PRAISE FOR *The*

"One of the finest experimental
will have a new generation of readers ducking its postmodern punches."

—Jane Marcus
Distinguished Professor of English,
The City College of New York

"*The Cook and the Carpenter* is particularly prescient in the context of
contemporary queer theory since, through its ungendered pronoun play,
the novel investigates the unstable categories of gender, sex, and sexuality. Bonnie Zimmerman's wide-ranging introduction usefully situates the
novel not only in the 1990's critical moment and in feminist political
actions of the early seventies, but perhaps most importantly, in Zimmerman's own emotional life as a lesbian scholar."

—Carolyn Allen
Associate Professor of English and Women's Studies,
University of Washington

"Arnold's book is mandatory reading for anyone interested in the literature and culture of the women's liberation movement. It has found a
worthy critic in Bonnie Zimmerman; her lucid and informative introduction illuminates both the historical and biographical contexts for the
book and the sources of its narrative power. Zimmerman explores the
intersections of literature, sexuality, and social change in original and
helpful ways. Thanks for the great read!"

—Deborah Rosenfelt
Professor of Women's Studies
and Director of the Curriculum Transformation Project,
University of Maryland

The Cutting Edge:
Lesbian Life and Literature
Series Editor: Karla Jay

Editorial Board

Judith Butler
Rhetoric
University of California
Berkeley

Blanche Wiesen Cook
History and Women's Studies
John Jay College and
City University of New York
Graduate Center

Diane Griffin Crowder
French and Women's Studies
Cornell College

Joanne Glasgow
English and Women's Studies
Bergen Community College

Marny Hall
Psychotherapist and Writer

Celia Kitzinger
Social Studies
Loughborough University, UK

Jane Marcus
English and Women's Studies
City College of New York and
City University of New York
Graduate Center

Biddy Martin
German Studies and Women's
Studies
Cornell University

Elizabeth A. Meese
English
University of Alabama

Esther Newton
Anthropology
SUNY, Purchase

Terri de la Peña
Novelist/Short Story Writer

Ruthann Robson, Writer
Law School,
Queens College
City University of New York

Leila J. Rupp
History
Ohio State University

Ann Allen Shockley
Librarian
Fisk University

Elizabeth Wood
Musicologist and Writer
Committee on Theory and
Culture
New York University

Bonnie Zimmerman
Women's Studies
San Diego State University

the
Cook
and the
Carpenter

a novel by the carpenter

JUNE ARNOLD

with an introduction by Bonnie Zimmerman

NEW YORK UNIVERSITY PRESS

New York and London

NEW YORK UNIVERSITY PRESS
New York and London

Copyright © 1973 by June Arnold.
Introduction copyright © 1995 by Bonnie Zimmerman.

All rights reserved

Library of Congress Cataloging-in-Publication Data
Arnold, June, 1926–
The cook and the carpenter : a novel by the carpenter / June
Arnold.
p. cm. — (The cutting edge)
ISBN 0-8147-0628-2. — ISBN 0-8147-0631-2 (pbk.)
I. Title. II. Series: Cutting edge (New York, N.Y.)
PS3551.R53C66   1995
813'.54—dc20   94-39793
CIP

New York University Press books are printed on acid-free paper,
and their binding materials are chosen for strength and durability.

Manufactured in the United States of America

10   9   8   7   6   5   4   3   2   1

Contents

Foreword

Despite the efforts of lesbian and feminist publishing houses and a few university presses, the bulk of the most important lesbian works has traditionally been available only from rare-book dealers, in a few university libraries, or in gay and lesbian archives. This series intends, in the first place, to make representative examples of this neglected and insufficiently known literature available to a broader audience by reissuing selected classics and by putting into print for the first time lesbian novels, diaries, letters, and memoirs that are of special interest and significance, but which have moldered in libraries and private collections for decades or even for centuries, known only to the few scholars who had the courage and financial wherewithal to track them down.

Their names have been known for a long time—Sappho, the Amazons of North Africa, the Beguines, Aphra Behn, Queen Christina, Emily Dickinson, the Ladies of Llangollen, Radclyffe Hall, Natalie Clifford Barney, H.D., and so many others from every nation, race, and era. But government and religious officials burned their writings, historians and literary scholars denied they were lesbians, powerful men kept their books out of print, and influential archivists locked up their ideas far from sympathetic eyes. Yet some dedicated scholars and readers still knew who they were, made pilgrimages to the cities and villages where they had lived and to the graveyards where they rested. They passed around tattered volumes of letters, diaries, and biographies, in which they had underlined what seemed to be telltale hints of a secret or different kind of life. Where no hard facts existed, legends were invented. The few precious and often available pre-Stonewall lesbian classics, such as *The Well of Loneliness* by Radclyffe Hall, *The Price of Salt* by Claire Morgan (Patricia Highsmith), and *Desert of the Heart* by Jane Rule, were cherished. Lesbian pulp was devoured. One of the primary goals of this series is to give the more neglected works, which constitute the vast majority of lesbian writing, the attention they deserve.

A second but no less important aim of this series is to present the "cutting edge" of contemporary lesbian scholarship and theory across a wide range of disciplines. Practitioners of lesbian studies have not adopted a uniform approach to literary theory, history, sociology, or any other discipline, nor should they. This series intends to present an array of voices that truly reflects the diversity of the lesbian community. To help me in this task, I am lucky enough to be assisted by a distinguished editorial board that reflects various professional, class, racial, ethnic, and religious backgrounds as well as a spectrum of interests and sexual preferences.

At present the field of lesbian studies occupies a small, precarious, and somewhat contested pied-à-terre between gay studies and women's studies. The former is still in its infancy, especially if one compares it to other disciplines that have been part of the core curriculum of every child and adolescent for decades or even centuries. However, although it is one of the newest disciplines, gay studies may also be the fastest-growing one—at least in North America. Lesbian, gay, and bisexual studies conferences are doubling and tripling their attendance, and although only a handful of degree-granting programs currently exists, that number is also apt to multiply quickly during the next decade.

In comparison, women's studies is a well-established and burgeoning discipline with hundreds of minors, majors, and graduate programs throughout the United States. Lesbian studies occupies a peripheral place in the discourse in such programs, characteristically restricted to one lesbian-centered course, usually literary or historical in nature. In the many women's studies series that are now offered by university presses, generally only one or two books on a lesbian subject or issue are included, and lesbian voices are restricted to writing on those topics considered of special interest to gay people. We are not called upon to offer opinions on motherhood, war, education, or on the lives of women not publicly identified as lesbians. As a result, lesbian experience is too often marginalized and restricted.

In contrast, this series will prioritize, centralize, and celebrate lesbian visions of literature, art, philosophy, love, religion, ethics, history, and a myriad of other topics. In "The Cutting Edge," readers can find authoritative versions of important lesbian texts that have been carefully prepared and introduced by scholars. Readers can also find the work of academics and independent scholars who write about other aspects of life from a distinctly lesbian viewpoint. These visions are not only various but intentionally contradictory, for lesbians speak from differing class, racial, ethnic, and religious perspectives. Each author also speaks from and about a certain moment in time, and few would argue that being a lesbian today is the same as it was for Sappho or Anne Lister. Thus no attempt has been made to homogenize that diversity, and no agenda exists to attempt to carve out a "politically correct" lesbian studies perspective at this juncture in history or to pinpoint the "real" lesbians of the past. It seems more important for all the voices to be heard before those with the blessings of aftersight lay the mantle of authenticity on any one vision of the world, or on any particular set of women.

What each work in this series does share, however, is a common realization that gay women are the "Other" and that one's perception of culture and literature is filtered by sexual behaviors and preferences. Those perceptions are not the same as those of gay men or of nongay women, whether the writers speak of gay or feminist issues or whether the writers choose to look at nongay figures from a lesbian perspective. The role of this series is to create space and give a voice to those interested in lesbian studies. This series speaks to any person who is interested in gender studies, literary criticism, biography, or important literary works, whether she or he is a student, professor, or serious reader, for the series is neither for lesbians only nor even by lesbians only. Instead, "The Cutting Edge" attempts to share some of the best of lesbian literature and lesbian studies with anyone willing to look at the world through lesbians' eyes. The series is proactive in that it will help to formulate and foreground the very discipline on which it focuses. Finally, this series has answered the call to make lesbian theory, lesbian experience, lesbian lives, lesbian literature, and lesbian visions the heart and nucleus, the weighty planet around which for once other viewpoints will swirl as moons to our earth. We invite readers of all persuasions to join us by venturing into this and other books in the series.

We are pleased to include *The Cook and the Carpenter* by June Arnold in our series of reprints. Not only was Arnold a novelist with a unique voice and innovative writing strategies, but with Parke Bowman she also founded Daughters, Inc., the 1970s publishing house of quality women's fiction. Together they published the work of Bertha Harris, Rita Mae Brown, Blanche Boyd, and other writers of note. It is this world where the gender of a writer matters that Arnold brings to her fiction. In a new introduction, Bonnie Zimmerman puts into perspective both Arnold and her engaging novel, *The Cook and the Carpenter*.

Introduction

Bonnie Zimmerman

There are points in a person's life that forever mark the divide between past and future. The ideas and experiences encountered then will have an impact far greater than might be understood at the time. One such turning point for me was the time period spanning from 1969 through 1973, an era that saw the emergence of the women's liberation and lesbian feminist movements. The ideas I encountered and the books I read then have had a greater effect on me than any books or ideas since. There were the foundational works of feminist theory like Shulamith Firestone's *The Dialectic of Sex,* Juliet Mitchell's *Woman's Estate,* Jill Johnston's *Lesbian Nation,* and, of course, Simone de Beauvoir's *The Second Sex.* There were the influential anthologies such as *Sisterhood Is Powerful* (Robin Morgan), *The Black Woman* (Toni Cade), and *Woman in Sexist Society* (Vivian Gornick). Most of all, there were the novels: Doris Lessing's *The Golden Notebook,* Marge Piercy's *Woman on the Edge of Time,* Isabel Miller's

Patience and Sarah, Alice Walker's *Meridian,* Monique Wittig's *Les Guérillères.* And there was June Arnold.

I encountered June Arnold's novels in 1973 as they appeared under the auspices of her own press, Daughters, Inc. First came *The Cook and the Carpenter,* then *Sister Gin,* and finally a reprint of her pre-women's liberation novel, *Applesauce.* I still have these, and a dozen other novels, in their handsome Daughters imprints on my bookshelves. June Arnold's writing has continued to resonate within me for the past two decades. As I began preparing this introduction, I came to realize just how profoundly she has influenced me. Not only have I written about her work as much as or more than any other literary critic, her words have provided the titles of two of my publications: " 'What Has Never Been': An Overview of Lesbian Literary Criticism" quotes from her 1975 speech at the Modern Language Association, and *The Safe Sea of Women,* a study of lesbian feminist fiction, draws upon a phrase in *Sister Gin.* I am truly one of June Arnold's literary daughters.

i

June Arnold was born June Davis on October 27, 1926, in Greenville, South Carolina, to parents who were both members of prominent southern families.[1] Arnold's father died when she was still a child, after which she moved to her mother's native Houston, Texas—a city and state that were to figure prominently in Arnold's novels, including *The Cook and the Carpenter.* In Houston, she enjoyed a life of privilege, including the best private schools, horseback riding, and, eventually, a first "coming out" as a debutante. After high school graduation, she attended Vassar for a year, but she missed the South and returned to Houston after only one year to finish her undergraduate education at Rice University. She married and had five children—one of whom died at an early age—and, at the same time, completed an M.A. in English at Rice. After divorcing her husband, Arnold moved with her children to Greenwich Village where she took writing courses at the New School. She published her first novel, *Applesauce,* in 1967. It was widely reviewed but generally misunderstood because of its experimental form and feminist content.

In the late 1960s, like many other women at the time, Arnold became involved in the women's liberation movement and came out for a second time—this time as a lesbian. She participated in the 1971 takeover of an abandoned building on the Lower East Side of Manhattan, an event that became the imaginative core of her second novel, *The Cook and the Carpenter*. After the takeover failed, Arnold moved to Vermont with her partner, Parke Bowman. In 1973 they used their own money to found Daughters, Inc., the first of the new women's presses to specialize entirely in novels. And what novels they were! Daughters published the early works of Rita Mae Brown, Bertha Harris, Elana Nachman (Dykewomon), Monique Wittig, Blanche Boyd, M. F. Beal, and June Arnold herself. Between 1973 and 1978, Daughters brought out eighteen novels and an anthology. Arnold not only was instrumental in publishing feminist fiction, she also strongly advocated the establishment of a separatist feminist publishing industry, arguing that "the first thing any revolutionary group does when taking over a government is to seize control of communications."[2] Arnold believed that writing and publishing were essential to a revolutionary movement; she argued that "women's presses are not an 'alternative'; they are in fact the real presses, the press of the future. Through them, the art and politics of the future are being brought to flower."[3]

In 1977, Arnold and Bowman tired of the harsh Vermont winters and moved themselves and the press back to New York City. The transition seems to have been fatal to their publishing concern, and in 1978 Daughters officially ceased to exist. Shortly after, the pair moved back to Arnold's home town, Houston, where she began work on her fourth novel, which was to be the story of her mother's life. Tragically, she was diagnosed with brain cancer shortly thereafter. Sonya Jones, an acquaintance, wrote later, "When told by her doctors she had a year to live, June Arnold reportedly responded: 'They've never dealt with a tough-minded woman. Darlin', let them hide and watch.' "[4] But not even she could tough out death, and on March 11, 1982, June Arnold died. Her final novel, entitled *Baby Houston,* was published posthumously in 1987.

The bare facts of biography cannot convey the totality of a life. June Arnold was a wise and witty woman whose life and work paint a complex portrait of the artist as feminist, lesbian, activist, publisher, mother, lover, and friend. She was an iconoclast and scathing ironist eager to proclaim her worldview at every opportunity. Her entry in a biographical guide to contemporary authors reads: "*Politics:* 'Feminist.' *Religion:* 'Women.' "[5] And, indeed, her work as a writer and publisher reveals her unbending commitment to promoting lesbian and feminist culture. There is no doubt that her early death robbed the women's movement and women's writing of a powerful force.

The vicissitudes of feminist publishing also robbed generations of feminists and lesbians of access to her fictional and theoretical writings. As Tee Corinne, with sorrow and restrained anger, points out:

> In 1985, three years after her death, many women attending the third *Women in Print* conference [the first of which Arnold had organized] in Berkeley, California, had never heard of June Arnold. Her books are out of print. Daughters, Inc., the publishing house which she co-founded along with her lover Parke Bowman, has ceased to exist. No one, to my knowledge is working on a biography. This is common within our movement, and it is a disaster.[6]

But time is beginning to mitigate the effects of that disaster. In 1987, her final novel, *Baby Houston,* appeared to wide and favorable reviews. The Feminist Press reissued *Sister Gin* in 1989.[7] And now, New York University Press is bringing back *The Cook and the Carpenter,* leaving only *Applesauce* currently out of print. In this way, we are piecing together the remnants of our history, so that new generations of readers will be able to discover the special quality of June Arnold's mind and art, while previous generations can reflect upon what we have lost. When contemplating her premature death, we should bear in mind the eloquent words spoken at June Arnold's memorial service: "They say that the moon is dead too, but still it gives light and makes darkness bearable."[8]

ii

June Arnold's critical oeuvre was small: one speech given at the 1975 meetings of the Modern Language Association and a dialogue with Bertha Harris, both reprinted in the special issue of *Sinister Wisdom* dedicated to lesbian writing and publishing; and a piece on lesbian publishing in *Quest*. Despite their brevity, her writings articulate a clear position on the political role of feminist literature. Arnold assigned to literature, particularly fiction, a privileged place in the feminist movement. The novel, she argued, "will lead to, or *is* revolution. I'm not talking about an alternate culture at all, where we leave the politics to the men. Women's art is politics, the means to change women's minds."[9] Like many of her contemporaries, Arnold deconstructed the opposition between private and public, or culture and politics, by arguing that women's literature, particularly the novel, could function as "an extension of and an intensification of consciousness-raising." Consciousness-raising was a mechanism through which activists in the early women's liberation movement created a collective view of reality. By drawing general conclusions from shared individual experiences, we found we could reshape and resist the assumptions and prescriptions inscribed within dominant discourses. Fiction, according to Arnold, could serve the same purpose, creating "a collective genius" or communal voice. In art as in politics, she notes, "we are all in the process of writing together."[10]

The first function of novel-writing as consciousness-raising, then, was to connect writers in a collective project. The second was to bring readers into the process. June Arnold, like most feminist writers and artists at the time, believed that cultural creation had an immediate and necessary effect on the consumers of art: "one of the lesbian writer's primary duties or tasks is to write in such a way that each woman reader learns to get in touch with her own source of truth."[11] In the post-poststructuralist nineties, it may be embarrassing to encounter words like "truth," not to mention "honesty" and "reality," which are also part of June Arnold's critical lexicon. These words belong to a theoretical perspective postulating that literature reflects or reveals a prelinguistic reality, so that by soul-searching the writer or reader discovers the authentic truth or real Self lying beneath the distortions of culture. To be sure, Arnold did believe in more or less truthful ways of depicting lesbian lives and, as a political writer, argued that fiction should give women tools for reclaiming and re-creating a different or, in her words, "very very heightened awareness of reality."[12] But her interest in and attention to the workings of language itself, and her belief in the value of literary experimentation, kept her from succumbing to the transparent realism that came to dominate lesbian fiction after the demise of Daughters. Moreover, Arnold's conception of self and identity was a precursor to contemporary postmodern theories. The truth that June Arnold pursued was the truth of her artistic vision; the honesty was her commitment to the story; the reality was what she called, after Gertrude Stein, "the infinite complexity of the present."[13]

Like many of her contemporaries, June Arnold's critical writing is replete with words like "new," "revolution," and "transformation." At that point in history artists and activists alike felt themselves to be involved in the creation of an entirely new world that would arise, like the phoenix, from the ashes of the old. *The Cook and the Carpenter* and *Sister Gin* embody this creative vision. Although received with respect, they did not make the kind of splash Arnold might have wished. Feminist publishing in 1973 was not as prolific and established as it was to become, and, existing as they did outside the mainstream, her later novels did not receive even the attention garnered by *Applesauce*. Only a small number of feminist and lesbian publications reviewed *The Cook and the Carpenter,* including *Ms.*, *off our backs,* and *The Village Voice* (this last written, with unabashed nepotism, by Bertha Harris). A handful of subsequent scholarly articles and books, including my own, address her writing in any detail. Significantly, many of these publications echo the refrain of "new literature," "new space," and "new lives" that we find in Arnold's own theoretical writing.[14] The lack of attention to June Arnold's work is partially explained, of course, by the collapse of Daughters as a publishing enterprise. But, in addition, I believe that June Arnold was too far ahead of her time and too idiosyncratic to be popular with either the mainstream or the lesbian reading public. She is an acquired taste, and like so many delicious things we learn to love, she rewards us with a deep and special pleasure.

The Cook and the Carpenter begins with three pieces of text that precede, and thus frame, the reader's entry into the story itself. First, the cover proclaims *The Cook and the Carpenter* to be "a novel by the carpenter"—a gesture that at once hides the identity of the author and exposes a seemingly naive identification between author and protagonist. (Amusingly, the entry on June Arnold in *Contemporary Authors* lists "Carpenter" as her pseudonym!) Although written in the third-person voice, it is portrayed as a first-person narrative. Apparently, we are to read the novel as the memoirs of its main character—who is June Arnold herself. But Arnold was too sophisticated a writer for us to take this identification seriously. Moreover, a reader familiar with the era that produced the novel ought to ask what gives the carpenter the right to shape these events into a story and define their meanings. Since the original action that inspired the story was non-hierarchical, and Arnold herself argued that women "are all in the process of writing together," shouldn't we reject the centrality and intentionality implied by the single, unified narrator?[15] Hence, in a clever move, Arnold undercuts her own identification of author with narrator by including a quote from the cook on the front cover as well: "I couldn't have said it better myself, though I would have said it differently." This wry comment subtly implies that *The Cook and the Carpenter* is about perspective and point-of-view, about who does and does not have the power to define, about established hierarchies and emerging equality. Each character has a particular slant on the events portrayed; the carpenter's—or Arnold's—story is only one among many.

The second framing device—the dedication "In Memoriam" to the Fifth Street Women's Building—identifies the novel as a tribute to a powerful moment in U.S. social history: the women's liberation movement. Built upon foundations at once feminist, socialist, and anarchist, the movement galvanized the energies of women across the country and from every walk of life. The movement attempted to tranform U.S. society at all its locations of power, including education, culture, language, politics, and the delivery of social services. Women all over the country began to establish women's centers. In New York City, for example, women from almost every women's liberation group took over an abandoned building on New Year's Eve, 1970—a symbolic date to be sure. As they wrote in the original mimeograph documenting the event:

> The purpose of the take-over was twofold: to dramatize the city's total disregard of the needs of the community (particularly women and children) and to let women know by our example that they can & must do things for themselves, and also to set up within a community (ours) and with the community of women themselves, services which are essential to our lives, run the way women know they should be run.

As the carpenter was later to say, they/we were trying to do two things at once, "set up a counterlife and work for a revolution" (50). In other words, through their action, they confronted the centralized authority of city administration and police and, at the same time, began to put into practice their vision of a revolutionary society. Their planned projects were all-encompassing and representative of the politics of the time (and the enduring needs of women): a food co-op, women's shelter, childcare center, health clinic, lesbian center, drug and alcohol rehabilitation program, and feminist school. A report on the take-over in *Rat,* a radical newspaper that itself had been taken over by feminists, lists "June" as the contact person for one more project, an inter-arts center.

The takeover was a huge success, attracting hundreds of activists and community members. It was ended by police action thirteen days after it began. As the novel depicts, the police reacted to the takeover with brutality and obscenities, while the women took every opportunity in jail and court to continue their consciousness-raising activities. Although some projects survived beyond the takeover itself, and meetings of the Fifth Street Building in Exile continued for some weeks after it ended, its most enduring legacy was June Arnold's *The Cook and the Carpenter.* In no small part due to the novel, the takeover acquired a legendary status in the history of the women's movement. The book stands as a monument to the politics and passions of the formative years of feminism, to its vision of a world in which women, "representing no specific group, and without any interest in pre-

iii

serving positions of leadership," could change the very foundations of society.[16] Hence, we can read *The Cook and the Carpenter* as an elegy not only to the takeover itself, but also to what it stood for: the hope that women working together could effect material changes in their own and other women's lives. If such change could not happen in "the real world," then it could in the alternate reality of fiction. From this action and its aftermath, we might conclude, June Arnold came to appreciate the power of the imagination and the way that literature could be revolution in itself.

Finally, the third of these introductory pieces of text opens up one of the most provocative aspects of the novel, June Arnold's creation and use of non-gendered pronouns. She introduces the story with an ironic epigram stating that, since gender differences are "so obvious to all, so impossible to confuse . . . it is no longer necessary to distinguish between men and women in this novel." "I have," she concludes, "therefore used one pronoun for both, trusting the reader to know which is which." Indeed, it is not until page 139 that gendered pronouns or single-sex proper names appear in the text. Prior to that moment in the story, Arnold uses invented pronouns—"na" and "nan"—as well as genderless proper names and titles to obscure the sex of her characters. (I should warn those who do not wish to have the "secret" revealed to postpone reading the rest of this introduction.) At the heart of the novel, then, is a mystery, the same mystery that was at the core of the women's movement: what is gender and why does it matter?

June Arnold was not alone in questioning the political implications of gendered pronouns. Feminists in the early 1970s cared very much about ridding language of its sexist elements. Before the advent of poststructuralist theory, Anglo-American feminists typically argued that language both shaped and reflected social norms; therefore, if we change the ways in which we speak and write, we can change society itself. Proposals to eliminate sexist language can be dated back to 1859. In 1970, Mary Orovan published a pamphlet proposing a generic pronoun, "co," that was actually used by alternative lifestyle communities. In 1973, the University of Tennessee tried generic pronouns in its student newspaper, but the experiment was dropped after only three months "in the face of misinterpretation, misunderstanding, and ridicule."[17]

If language in the real world was to prove so recalcitrant, fiction would prove more open to change. Marge Piercy, for example, used genderless pronouns in her 1976 utopian fantasy, *Woman on the Edge of Time.* Her experiment was less radical than Arnold's, since she employs her pronoun, "per," only in dialogue and does not introduce it until the reader has had time to adjust to the novel's terms and assumptions. June Arnold, on the other hand, cuts us no slack. She introduces her invented pronouns—"na" and "nan"—on the first page of the text, and sticks with them through dialogue and narration until the deliberate reintroduction of gendered language on page 139.

Discussion of these "pesky" pronouns dominates many contemporary reviews and subsequent readings of the novel. Each reviewer has her own theory about their meaning and impact. Are they a gimmick? Or is the reintroduction of "she" and "he" later in the novel the real gimmick? And, whatever one's conclusion, just what is the point? Is the pronoun "she" conferred upon the characters as an honor? Does the reintroduction of gendered pronouns illuminate the political dissension within the group? Or, as I have argued, does it reinforce the patriarchal authority of the police and judicial system?[18] I suspect such questions are not foremost in the minds of most readers, however. Whenever I have mentioned this introduction to friends, almost everyone has responded, "That's the novel with the funny pronouns, isn't it?" And too many have continued, "I just couldn't read it, you know."

There is no denying that the unfamiliar pronouns create an obstacle to smooth and easy reading. The eye cannot help but stop at the unexpected typography of each "na" and "nan," just as, in other texts, it fixates on misspellings and grammatical errors. A reader has to work at this book, has to want to make nan way through Arnold's dense web of ideas and imagery. But that, in part, was her purpose. According to her daughter, Kate Arnold, she believed in a "puritan work ethic": those pronouns were there to bring us to attention and to counter our lazy reading habits.[19] And indeed, June Arnold makes us work against the grain of all our complacencies.

For there is more than typography at work to disturb the reader's comfort. As Jan Hokensen, one of the few literary critics to pay serious attention to June Arnold's work, points out, without gendered names and pronouns we are unable to imagine the body; unable to imagine the body, we have difficulty relating to the subject or self:

> We scrutinize each character for gender clues ... knowing we should not need them but needing them desperately in order to apprehend "character" in any elemental way. We constantly apply to the text [critic Elaine] Marks's question about Colette's text, "is it female? is it male?" face to face with every shred of our own sexism."[20]

By undermining our expectations about gender, Arnold unsettles our notions about identity itself. If we are unable to determine if a character is male or female, we are forced to recognize that gender is not a biological essence, but a social construct. Moreover, the suppression of gender references results in a lesbian irony that challenges heterosexual assumptions: not only can women do anything, adopt any characteristic, act in any way — they can also love anyone, specifically, each other.

I can imagine June Arnold grinning fiercely in contemplation of her reader's terror as she or he takes up this challenge. After all, she had written that one of the lesbian writer's duties was "to experiment with the most direct, the most shocking, the most unpeeling kind of language to bring back this bond of communication [between author and reader], because this is going to be our only hope in the future."[21] Whether signifying gender, sexuality, politics, love, or parenting, her language is always of this "unpeeling" kind. I can also imagine with delight June Arnold's reaction to the anonymous professorial voice I recently heard echoing down the hallway: "These are the pronouns you may use: he, she, they, it."

iv

Over the past twenty years, I have read *The Cook and the Carpenter* several times, and each reading impresses me in a different way—no doubt because of my own personal and intellectual position at the moment. In one reading, I have marveled at June Arnold's depiction of radical political activity and discourse. In others, I have been intrigued by her characterizations, of the carpenter in particular, or by her dissection of the love affairs among the characters. In my most recent reading, I most often paused to consider how her text prefigures contemporary feminist theorizing over difference and identity. The following discussion will focus on just a few of the major themes of the novel, fully recognizing the untouched layers that each reader may uncover for naself.

The Cook and the Carpenter tells the story of a group of individuals who move to a small city in Texas to live collectively and create radical social change. The carpenter functions as the collective's "head" and conscience, the cook as its "heart" and feeder. As the novel opens, we watch these two characters move into an intricate sexual and emotional dance, sometimes together as lovers, at other times apart. The collective is rent by political divisions that eventually bring an outside organizer, Three, to Texas. The carpenter and Three become lovers, but find their union broken apart by the differences between them—just as the collective is unable to sustain its unity and cohesion. In part to mend these differences, they decide to occupy an abandoned building and turn it into a community center. As in the Fifth Street building takeover, they are busted after only a short occupation. The story concludes with Three moving on, and the cook and the carpenter reuniting and departing the collective.

The Cook and the Carpenter is about individual growth and change, relationships between lovers and between adults and children, and collective politics and social movements. In other words, it functions at the three narrative levels I outlined in my book, *The Safe Sea of Women:* the deliberate creation of new selves, new relationships, and new communities. It further portrays the breaking down of those structures—identity, couple, and group—through the interplay of difference amidst the presumed sameness of shared gender and political belief.

Within this story of personal relationship and political activism, the novel weaves a complex web of ideas and images. For example, it interrogates the concept of home in each strand of storytelling. Arnold moves the action from New York "back home" to Texas, in part because the loss of the Fifth Street Building—a political home—inspired her to return home imaginatively, to merge her personal roots with her newly acquired political identity. Hence, the carpenter tries to leave the "home" of her familiar identity and shape a new sense of self. The cook and the carpenter look to each other to establish the couple as home, but are impeded by the residue of patriarchal notions that continue to define for them the parameters of relationship. Finally, the collective struggles to create new definitions of family and home. Home, June Arnold suggests, is a concept and institution sorely in need of feminist transformation.

Although many particulars of human experience are portrayed in this novel—political activism and collective living, falling in love, being a parent, personal growth and change, ideological debates—certain concepts are woven throughout to create analogies, if not unities, among its multiple levels of narration. Its theoretical perspective is focused around the dualistic concepts underlying all social oppression and the dialectical struggle to transform them into new models for social change. Very early in the novel, the cook says to the carpenter, "It's about big and little, isn't it?" (10). If big stands for power and authority, and little stands for powerlessness and subordination, then indeed this novel is about big and little.[22]

The relationship between big and little resonates through the significant love relationships in the novel, those between the cook and the carpenter and between the carpenter and Three. The relationship between the titular characters is particularly interesting because it is here that Arnold challenges us most aggressively on our gender stereotypes. Without ever assigning her characters a sex, she plays with our tendencies to ascribe gender to certain human characteristics. The cook is little, poetic, imprecise, creative, flexible, a nurturer and feeder—in other words, "feminine." The carpenter is big, hard, intellectual, unyielding, detached, a shaper of wood—hence, "masculine." These stereotypes are reinforced (for some readers, presumably) by the characters' love for one another. Since the dominant framework is not only patriarchal, but heterosexual, one lover must be male and one female.

When, late in the novel, all characters are revealed to be women, our conventional assumptions about gender and sexuality are shattered.

As we can see, June Arnold anticipates some of the central insights of deconstructive theory that were to be introduced into feminism more than a decade later. Her concern is not primarily to invert dualisms, however, but to introduce a dialectical mode of thinking and being characteristic of the marxist discourse predominant in the early 1970s. Hence, into the original couple is inserted Three, the third term of the dialectic. At one time, the carpenter says, she had seen things "in pros or cons, this or that, a versus b—opposites." But Three introduces a way of being beyond dualisms: "you are all three at once—plus, minus and other. You are three if three is a perfect circle of all possibilities" (87). Three triangulates the relationship between the cook and the carpenter, opens up the struggle between the carpenter and Stubby within the collective, and introduces new feelings into the rigid mindset of the carpenter herself. Three is the principle of instability, of change and growth. She must leave at the end lest she become nothing more than one pole of yet another opposition.

These concepts—big and little, dualism and dialectics—are also at work within the novel's portrayal of political struggle. The collective is little in relation to the big forces of repression; its members must fight to establish their power as radical social activists. But more interesting are the dualisms, or differences, gradually revealed to be at work within the collective itself. There is currently a curious misconception that the early women's movement was oblivious to differences of race, class, age, or sexuality. The reissue of June Arnold's novels should demonstrate the inadequacy of that generalization. Arnold constructs a complex relationship between sameness and difference, unity and division. The collective at first focuses on what unites women, rather than on what divides them. But as these women come to understand that unaddressed differences of class, race, age, and political belief will fester and destroy their fragile community. Some collective members are "big" in relation to others: the carpenter, who exudes upper-class privilege and intellectual acumen, or Meredith who cannot recognize the children as unique individuals. Many pages of the novel are devoted to their struggle to name and reconcile their differences.

But Arnold gives an additional twist to this strand of storytelling: differences that loom so large in the minds of the collective are not recognized by the dominant society at all. To the police, for example, the women are all just commie dyke cunts:

> As they answered official questions, they were aware of the trivial nature of their own differences: whereas previously they had all felt that their group of women, coming together from different spheres, lives, ages, had meant that any conclusion the group reached had the validity of convergence, now . . . [t]hey were no more than a single gritty-eyed headache in the life of a giant. (139-40)

June Arnold intimates that "sameness" and "difference" are matters of perspective, not fixed states of being. Having begun with an unexamined belief in their similarity, the women of the collective believe they have worked through their differences to create a unity that is "a concentration, [a] force for change." In relation to the dominant structure, however, they lose the power of their diversity: "they had been rolled into one ball in order to be stamped out by one efficient foot"(140). From the conflict between sameness and difference emerges a synthesis, unity based on diversity. That forceful unity then must struggle with its opposite, the repressive power to flatten them into one uniform victim. The struggle between sameness and difference has no resting point, no ultimate conclusion; it constantly takes new shapes in response to changing local conditions.

The third strand of storytelling in *The Cook and the Carpenter*—that of growth and change within individuals—draws upon many of these same ideas. The titular characters both undergo changes that affect their relationship with each other and with the collective. The cook must become more independent and self-defined, which she does by baking a cake and eating it entirely—in other words, by producing and then consuming a symbol of her power and ability. The carpenter, on the other hand, must weaken, rather than strengthen, the walls she has built around her self. The carpenter exchanges her notion of identity as a unified, rigid "center," for one of fluidity, instability, and multiplicity. It is not incidental that the carpenter is a shaper of wood: her ego has been hard and unyielding as wood appears to be, but just as wood changes shape under the skillful hands of the carpenter, so too does the self prove malleable.

Several instruments are used to effect these changes: among them, love and sex, alcohol, and dancing. The carpenter has looked to her relationship with the cook and to communal living as means by which to dissolve the boundaries between self and other or intellect and feeling, but only when she falls in love with Three does she lose control over herself: "It was the carpenter's fantasy about naself, the one thing na most wanted to be—a non-be, in a sense; completely fluid" (86). She also looks for this fluidity in alcohol, one of the most controversial aspects of June Arnold's work. *The Cook and the Carpenter* is not as romantic about alcohol as is her next novel, *Sister Gin,* but it too valorizes drinking as a mode of liberation from fixed ideas, a way to blur the boundaries of self. But both novels also show the destructive consequences of unrestrained drinking. We cannot discount the impact of alcohol use and abuse in June Arnold's life and texts, but it would be unfair not to recognize the self-reflection and self-criticism present within the novels themselves.

Finally, I want to say something about the use of dancing in *The Cook and the Carpenter.* In the first chapter, we see a small child dancing like "a suddenly freed animal" (10). Throughout the novel, June Arnold uses dance as a metaphor for freedom, particularly from the rigidities and oppositions that keep individuals, couples, and communities locked up in prisons of past beliefs and feelings. The cook is able to let her body move and flow in dance, while the carpenter is as rigid in body as she is in mind. Through dancing, one dissolves boundaries, abandons the ego. Dancing also represents an interplay of instability and balance, which is played out in the transitory nature of the collective's political goals, the love affairs between the three main characters, and the carpenter's—or anyone's—identity. Through dance, we move from one place to another, all the while inscribing with our bodies the patterns of who we are. At the end of the novel, having gone through monumental changes, the carpenter returns to the cook—and feels like dancing.

I have been arguing that June Arnold anticipates the model of self—fluid, unstable, constructed by multiple discourses—that holds a privileged place in postmodern feminist theories. It stands in striking contrast to the essentialist Self that would emerge in later feminist and lesbian writing. But Arnold also anticipates the criticisms that have been raised against this notion of selfhood. What about those individuals for whom multiplicity may feel instead like fragmentation within a racist, sexist, and heterosexist society? Postmodern theory may underestimate their need for wholeness and harmony, torn as they are amidst the conflicting sites in which they must construct an identity. The character of Leslie, the only Black member of the collective and its most articulate lesbian voice, represents this point of view: "I feel like a tangle of bits of string.. . . I'm a fucking rat's nest of oppressed parts" (100). As the carpenter struggles against the uniformity within herself, Leslie—defined by very different social conditions—must work at untangling her bits and pieces of oppressed parts. Once again, Arnold asserts a complex, contradictory, and ultimately dialectical relationship between unity and diversity, sameness and difference, wholeness and fragmentation.

There is such depth and breadth in this short novel that a reviewer could point to any number of additional themes and issues for consideration. We might note, for example, Arnold's treatment of class issues within the collective and in the relationship between the carpenter and Three, or the powerful analysis of racism woven throughout the novel. Her dissection of political discourse is as skillful as anything written by our best political novelists, Doris Lessing for example. *The Cook and the Carpenter* is also masterful in its handling of children, both as individual characters and as points of contention within the collective. Arnold also makes insightful observations about the sexuality of mothers—the tension between nurturance and passion—and about what she called the "great untapped force" of power and violence within women.[23] I hope that this short introduction begins to suggest the range and quality of this extraordinary novel. *The Cook and the Carpenter* is a great achievement, one of the best fictional representations we have of the mood and daily activity of the moment in history that birthed feminism and lesbian communities. Welcome back after far too many years of absence.

Notes

1. I am indebted for biographical information to Linda Dunne's entry on June Arnold in *Contemporary Lesbian Writers of the United States: A Bio-Bibliographical Critical Sourcebook,* ed. Sandra Pollack and Denise Knight (Westport, CT: Greenwood Press, 1994), 31-36. Dunne very generously shared her notes as well as the finished essay.
2. June Arnold, "Feminist Presses and Feminist Politics," *Quest* 3, no. 1 (Summer 1976): 18. See also Lois Gould, "Creating a Women's World," *New York Times Magazine,* January 2, 1977, 10-11, 34-38.
3. Arnold, "Feminist Presses," 20.
4. Sonya Jones, "A Tribute to June Arnold: She Called Me Darlin," *Motheroot Journal: A Women's Review of Small Presses* 4, nos. 3-4 (Fall 1983): 1.
5. Christine Nasso, ed., *Contemporary Authors: A Bio-Bibliographical Guide to Current Authors and Their Works,* vols. 21-24, first revision (Detroit: Gale Research Company, 1977), 38.
6. Tee Corinne, "Remembering as a Way of Life," *Common Lives/Lesbian Lives* 19 (Spring 1986): 15. For another view of June Arnold and Daughters Inc., see Bertha Harris's introduction to her *Lover* (New York: New York University Press, 1993), xvii-lxxviii.
7. June Arnold, *Sister Gin,* with an afterword ("Under Review: How to Read a Hot Flash") by Jane Marcus (New York: The Feminist Press, 1989).
8. Personal communication, Roberta Arnold.
9. June Arnold, "Lesbians and Literature," *Sinister Wisdom* 1, no. 2 (Fall 1976): 28.
10. Arnold, "Lesbians and Literature," 29.
11. June Arnold and Bertha Harris, "Lesbian Fiction: A Dialogue," *Sinister Wisdom* 1, no. 2 (Fall 1976): 47.
12. Arnold and Harris, "Lesbian Fiction," 50.
13. Arnold, "Lesbians and Literature," 28.
14. Sam Stockwell, review of *The Cook and the Carpenter, off our backs* 4, no. 3 (Febrary 1974): 14; Annis Pratt (with Barbara White, Andrea Loewenstein, and Mary Wyer), *Archetypal Patterns in Women's Fiction* (Bloomington: Indiana University Press, 1981), 108; Melanie Kaye, "Lesbians and Literature," *Sinister Wisdom* 1, no. 2 (1976): 32.
15. Arnold, "Lesbians and Literature," 29.
16. *Rat* 18 (January 12-29, 1971): 3. Coverage of the police action is found in issue 19 (February 3-20, 1971): 5. The last mention of the Fifth Street Women's Building is in issue 20 (March 2-23, 1971): 20. Interestingly, *Rat* itself had been taken over by women from the male leftists who originally ran it.
17. Casey Miller and Kate Swift, *Words and Women: New Language in New Times* (Garden City, NY: Anchor Press/Doubleday, 1977), 118.

18. Bertha Harris, review of *The Cook and the Carpenter, Village Voice,* April 4, 1974, 36; Stockwell, review of *The Cook,* 14; Bonnie Zimmerman, *The Safe Sea of Women: Lesbian Fiction 1969-1989* (Boston: Beacon Press, 1990), 169.
19. Personal communication, Roberta Arnold.
20. Jan Hokenson, "The Pronouns of Gomorrah: A Lesbian Prose Tradition," *Frontiers* 10, no. 1 (1988): 67.
21. Arnold and Harris, "Lesbian Fiction," 48.
22. Bertha Harris makes this point in her *Village Voice* review.
23. Gould, "Creating a Women's World," 37.

the Cook and the Carpenter

1

"You know Texas. Do you think it's true?" the cook had asked an hour ago. The carpenter's answer was forgotten now in nan pursuit of truth: do I know Texas? Na surrounded this fact in the usual way: I was born of Texans and half-raised here—my second half, the older half, the half already halfway over into adulthood. The first half was reared in a deeper South where crops are grown and only livestock is raised.

From nan ninth to eighteenth year, the carpenter had lived in Houston. Nine years to know Texas, to absorb peripheral local color while one concentrated on the important thing: oneself. Nine years for Texas is a quarter-hour for every square mile. The carpenter knew na had foolishly wasted most quarter-hours on the same quarter-acres, not even counting the disproportionate time allotted to the milli-mile, nan bed; na had failed to prepare naself at all for the cook's assumption.

Na could say only that na knew quarter-acres of Houston, Galveston, Fort Worth; Sugarland and Sweet-water; Kemah, Corsicana, Amarillo; Edith, Alice, Beulah; etc. etc.—separate squares inside which na knew certain repeated figures of the patchwork quilt of unrelated pieces that was Texas: an expanse which agreed to act as a whole only where specific issues needed covering.

The land lay flat and silent, melted down from the few distant hills by a fierce August sun. The carpenter walked around to the east side of the porch and started the sander up again. I don't know Texas, but if "it" has the denier of violence, it probably is true. That thread joins cotton to calico in every state of the world.

The sander screeched across the worn boards, pulling up the patches of thick deck paint in gluey streaks, melting it, mixing the smell of burning lead and color into the air already thick with grit and dampness. The carpenter's breathing was protectively shallow. Na wore a strip of diaper around nan forehead to catch the sweat and prevent it from streaking nan glasses. The diaper was damp and now gritty itself and rubbed nan fore-head like a pumice stone.

Grit made na angry. "The woman is crazy," na said aloud. Or could be crazy. Therefore, na *could* be not crazy. Na cursed the circumstance that no one had heard nan story except the cook. They were planning to come Saturday, the woman said. It was now Monday. For almost a week life would stop before this threat, time disappear, all energy, thought and hope be thrust into planning how to deal with the careless violence of people unimportant to any of them. The carpenter wished suddenly that the warning had not come, thought suddenly that the warning itself was the evil, aiming to destroy them by detouring their lives into a week of reaction.

4

The stranger had come that morning at eight with a basket of eggs on nan arm and had walked straight up to the cook, announcing that na had brought the eggs (although no one had ordered eggs). They sat by the old icebox on the back porch, out of sight or earshot of anyone, and the woman told what na knew: that they were planning to come Saturday night.

"Will was serving at a party and the men were talking and laughing and carrying on about what they would do and all. Didn't take Will long to figure out what they was talking about, but na didn't let on na heard anything. Once one of them looked up and caught Will standing there wiping glasses and called out, 'Hey, Will, what you listening at over there?' And Will says, 'I want to beg your pardon, Mr. Jack,' and na walks over to the man, 'I'm sorry but what was it you said?' And the man says, 'What's the matter, boy, you getting deaf?' And Will says, 'Yessir, Mr. Jack, I've been having a lot of trouble with my hearing lately. I've got to see me a doctor.'

"When Will come home na told me what the men had said and all, and I told na there was nothing right about it and I was going to warn you folks over here. Na liked to have jumped out of nan skin. 'You say one word, girl, and I'll lay you upside the house lopsided,' and na come at me like a crazy man. I said, 'The side of this house is big enough for both of us, Mr. Williams, and I ain't afraid of you and I ain't afraid of those men neither.' Well, na hollered and cried and begged and called me baby and I said na was the baby and na didn't need to know every move I made noways and I come over here on my way to work."

The cook wanted the woman to stay and have coffee but na stood up and asked for a bowl to put the eggs in. "I'll bring you some more eggs towards the end of the week if I hear anything.

Right now I need a dollar for these."

"But what were . . . are the men planning to do?" the cook asked.

"Whatever it was last night, they're liable to think up eight different things by Saturday." The woman turned to leave. "Those kind got nothing to do but think."

The woman had walked then back down the driveway, carelessly holding nan empty basket, having stayed no longer than five minutes, just the right amount of time to make a usual delivery of eggs.

The cook described the incident four or five times, until all thirteen adults had heard it. There was no doubt in the cook's mind, one knew from the way na told the story, that na not only believed the woman but admired na tremendously. Yet the carpenter, listening in three different audiences, noticed that the cook varied the story slightly each time na told it. The woman's husband's name was different once, and the question of whether the woman's husband finally knew na was coming or whether the woman promised not to come and slipped out was unclear. When the carpenter questioned the cook on this point na grew exasperated and said, in the stubborn and poetic way the cook had, that it was the same thing either way. Besides, the cook had failed to ask the woman who the men were, their last names and the address of the house where the party took place.

"I believed na, that's all," the cook said, and then added, generously or sarcastically, the carpenter could not tell, "You would have too if you'd been there."

The carpenter stopped the sander to change its disk and relieve nan ears from the screaming assault of its ancient motor. Nan habit of mind during almost all of nan forty-three years was a balanced position between belief and disbelief, a harmonious central stand from which na could clearly see both the yes and the no, the + and the -, the danger and the danger. The carpenter did not like this quality in naself and sometimes

6

rationally chose to throw naself óver to one or the other side—not from belief or disbelief but from the need to belong or be other.

Hanging there like a beaded toy cat between brittle poles, like a child pulled on each arm by older friends going different ways, stuck like a nonswimmer between the wave that will grind you into the sand on its way to shore and the one that will break on your head, unable to hold only one belief at a time was to know fear very well.

The carpenter leaned all nan weight and muscle on the overheated sander and stripped the porch board by stroke. Na was anticipating grit in the cut shaped like an equal sign just off nan left eye and began to feel pain before it solidified. The eye throbbed. It was swollen and dark red in a neat ring.

The night before the carpenter had gone to a local bar with the cook. The carpenter had been feeling that expanse of the sometime drunk na expressed by the statement: These are our neighbors, we get to know them by drinking with them.

They were dull and easy with the fourth beer when a person sitting two stools down spoke to the carpenter. "I think you dropped your wallet."

The carpenter had seen the speaker come in, one of a couple dressed in the clothes of the town, whose round red face did not seem old enough to be topped with that thick white hair. The carpenter looked on the floor and then at the speaker.

"It looks like a wallet or a checkbook," the person said again. "There, under the stool."

The carpenter knew na had neither a wallet or checkbook with na. Na bent over to look once more out of politeness to white hair whatever its age.

"It's back there," the speaker said. "Farther."

The carpenter leaned over farther to peer into the dark floor under the cook's stool, and fell. Na hit the floor from stool height head first; with a thump na landed on the side of nan face by nan eye.

7

The bartender brought ice wrapped in a towel as if on signal. "Here. That's a nasty cut."

Two small gashes in the shape of an equal sign flanked the carpenter's eye where the hinge of nan glasses had been knocked into nan skin. The carpenter held the glasses now, one wire ear-piece jutting at a hundred and forty degree angle from the lenses.

The cook said, "Did na hit you?"

The carpenter shook nan head. "I lost my balance. I must be drunk." Na refused the ice-pack and ordered another beer.

The white-haired one smiled. "That's a nasty cut. You should put ice on it." No one said any more about a wallet or checkbook on the floor.

The next morning the carpenter had a black eye as perfect as if it had been socked with a fist.

It was the second black eye the carpenter had had since they had been in Texas. A week before a mosquito had sat on nan eyelid drinking its fill while the carpenter slept. In the morning nan lid was swollen and by noon the ring of dark red surrounded the eye.

Na attacked the splintered boards savagely, felt the abrasive diaper headband dig into nan forehead as if it wanted nan scalp itself. Last night's accident, na realized now, was caused by an agent no less deliberate than the mosquito. Na knew Texas too well to expect its people to be open except to each one's own class, race, sex, national and business equal. Others had to translate their own meanings from the doubletalk, flattery or sarcasm which was the rule. Straight language and level guns were no longer around when the carpenter had been young; now Texans had civilized themselves up to the practical joke, taken from animated cartoons.

The carpenter turned off the sander. Nan forehead was raw and the porch looked suddenly raw and beautiful. Na had gone to college and worked as a reporter in New York for fifteen years, being more careful than most to write down exactly what people said, in order to avoid having to decide what they really meant. Na stood under the outdoor shower for a long time, the cold water barely cool from the hot afternoon, until all the grit was washed away; then na went to find the cook.

Reporting, observing, recording, detached—the carpenter in nan earlier work had felt isolated most of the time, even though na had not clearly understood how isolated. Na had become a carpenter to become involved, to break away from detachment, not understanding at all how privileged being a carpenter was, or how the structures which were built by nan hands paralleled the structures previously set up in nan mind.

The scene in the huge backyard now under the long shadows of late afternoon was so alive and brilliant with late sunshine that nan heart suddenly skipped, jumped, hopped like a child eager to play. When na was a reporter, na had entered groups of people with pre-prepared anecdotes which na had waited a turn to tell, hoping to entertain and amuse or at least hold off feeling—which to na meant dissolving into the group and not, naself, existing. Now na watched still, hoping dissolvement would happen but painlessly, hoping na could just belong by being quietly there.

Andy (nan child) and two smaller children were building a treehouse. The carpenter walked toward them, stopped; na did not want to intrude adultness. Carter, who had been a laboratory technician last year, was playing a guitar to a circle. Carter sang in a voice as crisp and neat as the work na had once done. The carpenter stepped back, remembering that na naself could not carry a tune. The three who were called the theater group were laughing at each thing any one of them said. They lived in the rooms over the garage and the carpenter did not know them well. They were Meredith, Jesse, and . . . na could not remember the name of the third and did not join them. Na stood then at the edge of the backyard, nan heart regaining its own slow thump.

9

A small child, about three, was dancing a few feet from the carpenter, throwing nan body into the air and flinging nan arms in swoops. Na had only just come; the small group had arrived late last night from Pittsburgh. The blazing sun was low in the sky and cast huge dancing shadows in partnership with the child. Suddenly the child let out a high whine of fear; nan dancing, which had been that of a suddenly freed animal, became frantic. Na lept from foot to foot, immediately jumping off that foot and back to the other, crying now in terror. The carpenter instinctively looked over the grass at nan feet, expecting to see a small snake, bees, an anthill; when na saw nothing at all but grass and shadow na knew, lunged for the child and picked na up and held na high. The child was sobbing while the carpenter tried to explain then comfort na. Na had seen nan shadow. By picking up one foot na got rid of the huge unwelcome thing tacked on to naself, but when na put that foot down to free the other foot, the shadow caught na again. From foot to foot, na shook it off only to have it reattach itself. Na was as helplessly terrified as if na had been in quicksand.

The carpenter carried the child into the shade and found the cook and told na the story. "I want to tell you something else, too," the carpenter said. "About belief and disbelief. Last night, that person in the bar pulled the wallet trick deliberately so I would fall."

The cook stared; na laughed. "Of course. Na was little. Your weight falling, three or four feet—na could not have hit you so hard as na made you hit yourself: It's about big and little, isn't it?" The cook was little and the carpenter was big. Their own group was little and the men threatening to come Saturday were big. "Or we just assume they are big because we're used to thinking of ourselves as little," the cook said. "How do we know? There may be only three or four of them and we are thirteen not counting children. You know, I was thinking," the cook frowned. "That if that marvelous brave woman had not come to warn us, we would have spent this week doing something real for ourselves and what we believe in. And now we will all worry and discuss and plan, instead, how to deal with *them*. They got control of us, just like that."

"You know, that's exactly what I was thinking a while ago."

"We could go one step further," the cook said. "And be you in the bar last night—do exactly what we would have done in the first place."

"Ignore them."

"Make them not exist." The cook laughed. "Even though they do."

"I guess they do. You believed na, anyway."

"Na was too real not to believe."

"So are you," the carpenter said.

The cook pulled out a cigarette and offered one to the carpenter, who shook nan head. "Am I the only one here who's still smoking? I knew I'd get some distinction if I just kept on smoking—if you just keep on doing one thing long enough . . . Sure, I'm so real I called my own child a son of a bitch this morning. Na kicked the baby in the face and said, 'I'll kill you in your sleep.' Or maybe it was because na was throwing peas at my face pretending they were bullets."

"Maybe just because na was throwing food."

"I said, 'Why you son of a bitch!' and slapped na as hard as I could. It was ten minutes before I realized what I had called myself, in that case." The cook lit the cigarette and looked across the yard into the distance, nan face in the shade as solid and marked as if it had been carved out of wood, enduring for centuries. "We're afraid of each other, too, all of us. Not just you."

"You?"

"We're afraid another person might see into us and not like us if we're not liking ourselves just then, or that they might be envious and attack us when we're liking ourselves too much. Or maybe it's something else. But we're all afraid; I know because I am. It's

11

what keeps us working so hard." The cook stood up. "I have to go do dinner. Come too."

"I've never made chili before," the cook said, turning on a low fire beneath the restaurant-sized pot. Na went to the radio sitting on a shelf of clutter, found a station playing Mexican music, listened a moment then turned the volume high. Na began to sway and then dance, stepping in half-arcs back and forth and snapping nan fingers. "As soon as we get the feel of it, we can taste it," na said, laughing but far away, nan black eyes growing Spanish and olive. The carpenter tapped nan feet too and yielded to tiny steps. The cook tasted, added chili powder, and switched to a livelier dance as the music changed. An undersized, lithe, almost child-like figure, na moved to an internal primitive rhythm, parent and child as one, twisting through the holes of parenthood and leaping around the borders of the child, stopping only to taste, add, taste, enjoy, taste. The carpenter saw the possibilities of moving too; with a timid laugh, na stepped out, and turned, and stopped to taste . . .

"I really don't think it's fair to the children to keep them waiting for dinner just because you feel like dancing." The voice from the doorway was strong and clear and the carpenter stood still, automatic instant response. The cook turned once more away from the figure in the doorway and, turning back, bowed obsequiously.

"The children, of course," na said in a honeyed voice. "How could we forget the children?—whom we live for every precious minute unless we're hideously selfish."

"It's not fair to the rest of us at all," the voice in the doorway backed down. "It's hard enough to live to-gether without some people going off on ego-trips."

"Or it's delightful to live together and allow us fucked-up freaks our silly little ego-trips," the cook said.

12

"All right, let's talk about that." The figure moved into the kitchen and sat down. Na was a social worker and political organizer from New York, had been for twenty years; na was tough, old, efficient, well-organized and certainly brave. Na was called Stubby because nan last name was Stubbs, but the carpenter could not use the name without guilt. It fit so well the blunt body and foreshortened outlook of the person it referred to that the name came too close to description to pass as an accident of lineage.

"You tell everyone in the group that a gang of crazy people are coming after us Saturday night," Stubby said, "and everyone spends the day thinking about that and planning to talk about it in the meeting tonight, while you go dancing around as if you didn't even take it seriously. The least you could do, it seems to me, is help us get dinner over with and start the meeting so we can get through with it before midnight."

The carpenter saw Stubby's broad back and the lines on nan face which described twenty or more probably forty years of fighting and learning to fight and win, and knew that if the men did come Saturday they could all depend on na. The cook saw it too; nan eyes grew calm and na said, "I'm sorry."

"You have to take these things seriously," Stubby said and got up and left.

The cook laughed and danced a last few staccato steps, snapping nan fingers over nan head: "Bu-bu-bu-bu-bu-lllllll-sh-sh-sh-shhhhhhh . . ."

The carpenter felt the wave of joy of the cook's laughter and then the equal crash of nan own guilt: that na could feel joy at Stubby's being put down (the sterling values of work for others and seriousness above all), and guilt that na could still feel such guilt (the rejected values of guidance counsellors and advisors above all). Na could even

13

feel guilty that na felt guilty for feeling guilty. Na saw that the cook, as nan Mexican self at least, lived far beyond such gloom and sogginess; the carpenter then knew the envy that closed its claw around nan heart like ice.

2

The two young people bent over the machine, their heads like shining parentheses enclosing a tape recorder.

Chris turned off the machine. "Why don't we summarize that we have three choices: run away, call the police, meet the attack in some way. No one wants to run away . . ."

"No one says na wants to run away," Andy said.

"Right. And everyone thinks that even if we call the police we will have to be prepared also to meet the attack, because they won't come until a crime is being committed."

Andy wrote it down. "That's the easy part of the summary."

"And then we list all the suggested ways we could meet the attack."

Andy wrote: guns, bodies, bottles and clubs, dogs, barricade, or reasonable persuasion followed by etc.

15

The day was hot and na wanted to go swimming. Na was fifteen and had expected that the job of writing up the minutes of the meeting would take less than an hour, but they had been here already two and a half. "Don't you get tired of meetings where nothing is decided?"

Chris was seventeen, although na was no taller than Andy. "Most people—in this country; I can't speak for the world since I don't know most people in the world—only fight when they feel threatened," Chris said.

"Even if that's true, what about the others?" Andy said.

"The books are never about *them*. But if the first statement is true, we should find out why these men feel threatened and explain to them that they're wrong to feel threatened, etc.—whether they are or not, of course."

"Yeah. That won't be as much fun as just fighting back. I'd really like to hit them."

"Bored with the revolution? Well, in that case, the cook's idea would be the next most fun. Do you think you could pretend that you were crazy?"

"I don't know, Chris. I haven't been sane yet." It was a statement of fact and Andy's fluid face took on a sudden angular unanimity, foreflash of an adult.

Chris nodded. "We're lucky."

"I forgot to feed the chickens!" Andy suddenly ran out.

Chris took the notes back to the room na shared with Leslie, to write them up. Leslie was crouched over a frame of two by fours on the floor. Na was building a partition, a room divider.

"You really want to cut this poor little room in two and keep the north and the south from even talking to each other?" Chris said.

Leslie spoke around the nails in nan mouth. "What are you, some kind of liberal?"

16

"How do I know I'm going to have as much light over here as you have over there?" Chris said. "I've heard that separate but equal sequel before. It means you think I'm a sloven."

"Of course I don't. I think you keep your clothes on the floor so your feet will have something soft to walk on. I think you don't wash your sheets because you don't want to pollute the nation's water supply. And I know you keep all that garbage around because mice aren't eligible for food stamps."

"You think I have wonderful qualities—earthiness, simplicity, goodness with children and animals."

"The entire room owes you a debt which we can never repay." The noise of the electric saw filled the room as Leslie got ready to cut four diagonals. One bare foot held one end of the two by four down, the other end was braced against the door molding. Leslie bit nan lip and inched the saw carefully down the pencil line. When na had cut the fourth line na released the "on" button, put the saw down gingerly and wiped nan face. "It doesn't matter that you'll never be able to handle the big dangerous tools we use. You have your own quaint ways of doing things—like that curtain you put up to divide the room, that kept falling down every night."

"I add flavor. I'm spontaneous. I laugh a lot."

"You can dance."

"You'd just rather not share a room with me. Because I'm really a dirty slob who'll be happier with my own kind."

"We can visit." Leslie tried to hold the diagonal across the corner of the frame and nail it at the same time. It kept slipping. "You can help me hold this piece of wood now if you want to."

Chris knelt on the floor and pushed the wood-brace into the side pieces. "I can visit you?"

"If you think you'd feel at home in my room." Leslie hammered one nail in. "Course you might feel more at ease if I visited you."

17

"Will you be bringing a basket?"

"Well, knowing how much you like candy . . ."

"Am I going to have to start liking whiskey now that I'm seventeen?" Chris said.

"Okay, let's stand this thing up—where the pencil mark is." They raised the partition-frame almost upright. It stuck on the ceiling about fifteen degrees short of the perpendicular. "I couldn't have measured it wrong," Leslie said. "Push." They pushed; it moved less than an inch. "I know I measured it right. I did it three times."

"We don't have to hold it any more," Chris said, letting go. "It's stuck."

"Do you mind if the wall slants a little?"

"Since it's slanting into my half, it must be what I deserve."

"Maybe if we hammer both sheets of plywood onto your side, the hammering will move it some more."

"We could hammer one sheet of plywood and then just hammer the frame," Chris said. "Otherwise I won't get any shelves."

"They're only two-inch shelves."

"One and five-eights inches."

"Uppity. Sassing your betters."

"Give us two inches and we'll take an inch and five-eights. We're slipping backwards. It's those equal schools you set up everywhere."

Leslie sat on the bed, nan dark eyes suddenly serious. "Are you going to go to school next month?"

There was only one high school for the town, a huge glass and concrete structure on the other side of Main Street which they had visited the week before. Leslie had dressed with care for the day, choosing clothes from the group's supply which were nearest like those na had seen the town's teenagers wear. Chris, whose life to now had been spent in New York City's progressive private schools, refused to make any concession beyond wearing clean bluejeans and a clean shirt, both patched.

18

There were people at the summer-school session dressed like each of them, people with hair like theirs, who walked like they did, whose faces were as open—but they were a small handful and had apparently had no influence on the meticulously-ordered chill of the school. Every bulletin board and blackboard bore out the impression of hierarchies and organization and expertise. Chris flatly said na would not go to the school. Leslie wanted to go but not alone. They had argued energetically; neither side budged.

"Look, I've thought about it since we visited," Chris said now. "I'll go if you still want to."

"I sure do. I want to at least graduate from high school." Leslie laughed. "I used to want to be a lawyer, before I decided to be a criminal instead."

"It'll be a way of meeting the people around here, I guess. Andy'll have to go anyway." Chris stood up. "But I don't look forward to it. They don't even play soccer down here. But like our president, I'd do anything to achieve peace and quiet. Let's finish this insulting wall of yours."

At five o'clock the carpenter found the cook on the back porch. Na was playing a game of chess with a child named Nicky, a skinny child with eyes so bright they looked wet and a pointed face like an elf—the cook's second child, the one na had called a son of a bitch.

Nicky looked up and grinned at the carpenter. "I always win," na said.

The carpenter's own children, now almost grown, had been raised mainly by others. "Are you that good?"

"I'm the best!"

The carpenter waited until the game was over.

"I won, I won!" Nicky threw the words at the carpenter's face like the peas of yesterday. "I told you I always win!" Na ran into the yard to tell the other children.

"Does na always win?" The carpenter tried to remove the disapproval from nan voice.

19

"Na can't bear to lose," the cook explained to the disapproval nevertheless. "I know because once I won and na cried and screamed for an hour."

"Shouldn't na learn that na can't always win?"

"I don't know. I learned that the price of my winning was to deal with a tantrum for an hour."

"But the older children—do they treat na like that?"

"Well, at first they beat na, they would win of course. But then when na cried they didn't do it again. They learned not to."

"So Nicky is learning to cry to get nan own way."

"Na is learning that if something upsets you so much that you have to cry and you let your friend know that, the friend will be able to understand and comfort you. Na is learning to communicate."

The carpenter was polarized into silence and felt one-directional and simple as an adult; the cook was child, knew child, created naself the mind which the child did not know it had.

Two years ago na had seen the cook at a school fair in New York City and that first impression, like a footprint on the mind, remained over the carpenter's eyes as a frame through which all subsequent encounters with the cook were seen.

At the fair was a "night club"—the science room decorated with an astronaut motif and adult alcohol—and the carpenter had retreated there to recover from the dual torment of being a parent and social conversation. The group at the table next to na dominated the room—their laughter defined laughter and rendered tin the noise and vague touchings at other tables. Dominating the table itself, carrying its rhythm, was the cook.

At first the carpenter saw only wild dark hair and the kind of arresting face rarely seen except on a baby animal, which unlike the baby animal's moved and shifted through so many circles of joy that the carpenter felt kaleidoscopically hypnotized. Na sat and stared, cold and blond as if na wore the armor of the northern church.

20

Suddenly the cook stood up and began moving to the tame music of the science room as if na were on a mountain. The rest of the parents turned to watch and the hired combo—three father-like figures—limped their instruments, watched and picked up then with a new rhythm being conducted by the dancer.

It was a dance of the body in moonlight, awkward sweeping into a leap of grace, heaviness failing to soar turning into a spin of air and back to earth: a dance that said, I the dancer deny that I am dancing do not laugh my body is struggling to evaporate. The carpenter's mind detached itself and broke free to be swayed and tossed as it floated over the dancer.

Flushed and abruptly finished, the cook sat down and looked suddenly like a forty-year-old inhabitant of New York, cynic repudiating the gypsy.

The image that remained in the carpenter's mind, although fixed in detail, was principally one of motion as if the skin itself were fluid and the whole so unstable that the eye had to catch it like the pattern of a cloud. The carpenter's own face—chiselled, patrician, frozen in middle-age—stared back from any mirror like a fact.

Suddenly now under the wide outgoing Texas sky at the immense hour of five-fifteen, the carpenter felt something rustle and threaten to explode inside na; it was the urge to throw naself, the fact, into the maelstrom of the cook's heaving ocean and bob there, in the most extended position possible for a fact, until na was shredded loose.

Na reached for the cook and hugged, holding gently as a delicately-balanced beach ball, holding the need to touch, dizzy and barely breathing with nan eyes closed into that dark spray of hair. Na felt the cook's hand press against the back of nan head. The carpenter said, at last, after two years, "I love you."

That night during the second meeting to discuss how to deal with the Saturday night attack, the carpenter for the first time sat unmoved by the fact that everyone

21

else easily said, This is how I feel . . . , whereas na naself spoke only from the icy determination of the tongue-tied. Tonight the carpenter sat by the cook, tingling, vibrating, softened all over by the extraordinary words na had said earlier; I love you. Na did; na had for months. The group disappeared and had no more the power to intrude than images on a screen to the couple blanketted in one seat watching.

Then the cook spoke. "Something really beautiful happened to me this afternoon, something I want to share with the group. A person I've known and loved as a friend for two years did something that took more courage than I have—we all know how afraid we all are of being rejected. This person came up to me and said, 'I love you,' meaning 'in love.' Because na had the courage to grow."

The carpenter's ears felt boxed with echoes. Na heard nan own sacred urgent embrace coupled with the story of the child who cried to announce that nan need was to win, and both things described by the phrase, "guts to take a new step." A hundred miniature alarms ringed the carpenter's brain.

"So should we as a group," the cook explained. "Be able to seek out our own growth."

Then through the ringing one word came clearly, "mind." The carpenter shook nan brain to dismantle the clocks and .listen; the cook's voice was pointing at the carpenter's head and was hoping that the other person did not mind na (the cook) saying this, that na (the cook) was sure the other person (now clearly the carpenter) did not—"none of us came all the way to Texas to protect our privacy, the one thing we all know kept us locked up in the hope chests of the system back there."

The cook then outlined a plan for Saturday night, that they have a happening, a carnival with theater and poetry and music and invite everyone in the neighborhood and reporters and the mayor; that they use it as a way of reaching out to the community even though they had only been here two weeks and were not really ready for that and shouldn't expect . . .

The carpenter heard almost nothing of the plan or the excited discussion which followed, most of it in favor. Na was trying to retrieve nan politics which tumbled across the floor of nan mind like a barrel of puppies overturned and changing directions faster than the hand could react. A giant tear lodged in nan throat, focussing nan mind back on naself, forced naself back into the child who still believed that one thing could be true and who had to stand in a circle of fingers pointing at proof that it was not.

Certain structures would need to be built and there was not much time. The carpenter was being asked a question. Nan eyes were deep-set behind glasses, which recessed and veiled their pain into unnoticeability; na knew that and looked straight at the questioner's face. Of course na would. Begin first thing in the morning . . .

After the meeting the carpenter, no longer feeling like the carpenter, thinking of naself simply as small child grown into the usual prison, unable to grab even a single political puppy, listened to the people who wanted to do theater describe what they wanted . . . suffocated, watched the cook surrounded by others, felt the room fill with a closeness, a sense of being united which they had not shared for days. The eyes of one of the people talking to na now sought nan's . . . to congratulate na? Na felt there were too many others. The carpenter sought a corner. "Can we discuss it over here?" It was too close. "Let's go outside . . . "

Na waited for the cook and longed for a drink of gin.

Walking toward the brook which sliced off their northern corner, the carpenter's hand reached for the cook's, drew back. Na felt confusion pounding nan head as if each separate part of nan brain were swelling up against its neighbors. Nan skull would hump up in the middle like a Texas sidewalk in the heat if na could not pour gin between the pieces and quiet them.

"Look. I feel all those things you said we don't feel

anymore," the carpenter said.

The cook was floating bare brown feet in a trickle of water. Na looked at the carpenter's face, nan own a foot away. "So do I," na laughed.

The carpenter's hand reached into the cook's hair, long curved fingers cupping nan skull as if it were most fragile wood, carving so covetted nan hand trembled. Confusion raced from nan brain as na held nan lips gently over the cook's mouth and nan breath stopped and they kissed. The cook's body like flesh made fur softened the carpenter into simplicity. The intricately-structured interiors of nan past screamed and exploded; glinting poles of color appeared in their place. Na stared at the cook's face and knew that na was feeling love for the first time—love without fear or craft or division.

"I don't hear any voices," the cook whispered. Crickets and leaves and the brook's game with its pebbles and their own breath and motion surrounded them, but that was outside; inside was silent. "I've never kissed anyone before except in the presence of thoughts in words. A thousand comments. Do this. Think this. What if . . . .? What are you doing? My mind is six hours old." A frog croaked and na smiled and grew serious. "I've never done this before."

On the damp dark earth smelling of summer and insects, the carpenter felt nan nose fill with the smell of the cook's face and nan mouth with the tang of saliva; nan hand on the cook's chest tingled. "Are you sure you want to do it in private?" na whispered.

The carpenter took off nan shirt and the cook's bluejeans and put the shirt under na bare skin and nan own hand ached when it touched na. They stroked each other's skin and the palms of their hands were stroked back by the skin. They tasted each others mouths for a long time. The cook bit the carpenter's neck and pulled back and bit again and said, I'm sorry and I can't help it and bit na again and cried out and the carpenter's own orgasm shook nan whole body a moment later.

A sudden rain made the leaves over their heads flap

and the sound of the rain reached them before its wetness. They licked the water from each other's faces, "God thinks sex is dirty," the cook said.

"Na doesn't. That was applause. Didn't you hear it?"

"Your face has changed," the cook said. Na stopped at the edge of the trees and stared at the face of a friend two years, now lover. "It's new. Has mine?"

"Yes, but it doesn't matter. You've already told everyone anyway."

"You did mind."

"I felt used."

"Really? But I think it was important for you." The cook kissed the hand na was holding. "Everybody loves the baby when you take off its diaper."

Like most cooks, the cook was also a painter. Na lay awake now in the carpenter's single bed, propped so that na could see one tree in the moonlight. The tree reminded na of nan body. Na did not paint trees, but na had painted nan own body dozens of times. The tree was squat with spreading branches, a mimosa in scattered late-summer bloom, feathery not solid, and uneven. Na had painted nan body, often backwards, as if it were body—shape outlined in a stingy few lines, often close to commercial art (nan training). It was the body of being human which no human being would want.

Na remembered a pornographic film na had seen, had been socially forced to sit through in high school by a group of peers. The cook had immediately detached naself (symbolically) from these now so-called peers and had determined to get something different out of the film than what they got or expected from na. The film was of six naked people making love with people of either sex or themselves. The cook was sixteen. It was easy to avoid being shocked. It was less easy to avoid laughing because although there was panting and moaning and grimace, nothing happened on the bodies; nothing erected, changed color, throbbed or pulsed. Then one body responded, one out of six. The camera

25

zoomed in. The cook's mouth quickened, nan own sex swelled up and pushed against nan heart. The expeer group was supposed to finish off the film by trying to have an orgy. The cook went into the bathroom instead, locked the door, took off nan clothes and balanced on the edge of the bathtub to look at nan body, sections alternating, in the medicine cabinet mirror. My body is beautiful, na decided for the first time since na was five; it is just like the body on the screen which responded.

In the years that followed, the only consequence of the mind's decision that day was subsequent decisions. No feeling of beauty had grown, only isolated instances of receding inadequacy.

Until tonight. Now nan body felt extraordinary, the sense of feeling focussed on nan palms as if one first experienced the metaphor literally. Na stroked nan skin from neck to hip, each pad of flesh feeling alive into its deepest layer, each layer connecting to its neighbor, each surface retaining the stroke after nan palm had passed as if its aliveness existed independently and merely needed to be called up.

Na stared at the half-hidden sleeping face of the carpenter.

The next morning, building the simple platform and complicated frames and sign-backings the happening required, surrounded by various members of the group at different times, the carpenter felt again that na was being congratulated. The cook's disclosure of nan most personal (because it was uttered at the instant it was felt) declaration of love had made the carpenter suddenly popular. And uneasy. Na smiled a lot.

Na did not hear voices anymore either. Na heard jargon. Na heard phrases which had been substituted for in nan mind by letter and number combinations—a person spoke, ping, the formula flashed across the screen and the lower right hand light announced it correct. What was Chris saying? The young people were enjoying themselves in the sunshine, preparing for a party. Chris . . . nan child? Seventeen, and knowing what now with which to mock nan parent? Na will never be tall and does not mind. Na laughs but never smiles, at home in sunshine. Na looked into nan parent's eyes once; knew na well enough not to press, looked away. But the others who were in love acted as if na was one with them. Animal leveller. Someone was going to touch na, hug na, feel nan body stiff and clinging to privacy.

Na pretended to be working very hard. Na frowned and looked down a length of two by four, bent to look at an imaginary space, took out a pencil and alternated looking and noting down numbers. Na was absorbed in a difficult problem. The others respected nan preoccupation or were themselves coincidentally preoccupied; na was alone. The air just over nan body surfaces skinned quickly. Nan hearing dulled. Na saw only the two by four and numbers. For a few seconds na breathed deeply and freely, until the skinning was complete; then the surface hardened further and na was enclosed and could not breathe at all.

Safely shut up, na thought of the cook. Nan body shuddered as if underneath a ferryboat engine were reversing itself; na refelt the cook's touch on nan skin and grew dizzy, daylight vanished, na hung in a vibrating cocoon of black and felt na would faint, not from lack of real air but from the close breath of last night's memory swaddled up in there with naself.

"We're going to lunch." The voice outside had the metallic quality of a voice repeating the words a second time.

The carpenter juggled the figure into focus: Chris, whose grey eyes, like most of the grey eyes of nan generation, inspected every visible thing for traces of phoniness. Na could look at nan parent steadily waiting for an answer to lunch, and search: is it possible for one's parent to be in love and what does it feel like from that height and thinness of passion?

27

The carpenter had kept all but the primmest manifestations of nan love affairs from the children—they knew the verbal justifying of relationships and an arm over a shoulder. Feeling, the expression of which was the obscenity of the fifties, was kept for closets along with discussions of money. The carpenter was embarrassed now and spoke of lunch; defying embarrassment then, na said, "Do you like the cook?—or whatever word you use for 'like.' "

"Sure." The monosyllable was flat and ambiguous. "Andy wants to know if you mean love or the other kind of love."

"Both." The carpenter, relieved to be handed a four-letter answer, put a hand on nan child's silken scrambled hair and touched with a kind of tender awe the possibilities of seventeen. "It may seem strange to you, but I think it's the first time in my life when both kinds of love have been together for me. It has a lot to do with the people here, with being here . . . I think I've changed."

"I think so too."

"You think you have or I have?"

"Oh, I change all the time; *we* all do." Na meant children as opposed to parents and the carpenter felt slapped into a leftover. "I meant I think you have." The steadiness of Chris's revolutionary grey eyes made it seem that na was on the point of accepting nan parent as a "we." "Of course it may not be a real—lasting—change." The revolution gives and takes away.

"It is," the carpenter said from a parent-past, simultaneously realizing that nan tone denied it. "I know it is," nan voice was soft, "because every part of me feels it—my hair, throat, fingernails, knees—especially knees—and belly. Let's go to lunch. I really love na." The carpenter felt stranger than na had ever felt in nan life, saying that to nan child—not reporting a fact, but feeling what na said as na said it. "I guess it's good that you knew from the beginning, because otherwise I would have spent weeks not telling you."

28

Chris walked with nan hands in the pockets of cut-off jeans and nan head studying the ground. "It's okay for me but Andy . . ." Na looked at the profile of nan parent. "Andy thinks you should have told us yourself."

In the carpenter's mind the scene expanded: na would have told them, in a week or two, month or two—told them during a walk in the fields or behind a kitchen table, all their attention directed at their remaining parent, all their awe focussed on . . . a parent with a self of its own. And all three of them could wonder how it would affect the children. Triangle behind the kitchen table; apex: carpenter. Na had never been able to do anything without deciding how it would affect someone else so that the someone else's reaction became the life of the thing done. Or because drama had for so long been a thing in books that to stage nan own situation with a real audience left na trebly alive. Or because na had too often been the reactor of others, to be the cause was the sweetmeat. No. Because na alternated between being a rubber raft on sea waves and refusing in terror to be that, na only felt peace when na was the one who launched the raft in the first place. One-third of naself winding up the other two-thirds. Initiator or confused.

"I didn't have a chance," the carpenter said and laughed.

Chris's answering laugh was as startling as a fish jumping clear of the water. "I guess Andy can understand that," na said.

3

The night of the carnival the carpenter was the only person from their group who was not happy. From nan own nature na had doubts; when these were not shared by anyone else, they increased and throve in an open field. On everyone else's face, excitement reigned over a terrain reaching from pleasure to hysteria.

The cook was close to the latter border. Na had not only conceived the original idea; na had also done most of the detail work. Na had made each person a vest which slipped on over the head, giving a panel of cloth covering the chest and back. On each panel was painted, YOU, in large letters of red or orange or black or blue or green. By now all the children and most of the adults had one on, so that everywhere the carpenter looked na saw, YOU, which had an unsettling effect upon nan need to be separate. The carpenter thought therefore that the vests were silly, and doubted that

30

they would unsettle strong and determined madmen at all.

There were no madmen present anyway; the only community people attending the carnival were parents bringing a child or more, who wandered confused over the front yard looking for cotton candy and the usual games that the word carnival had led them to expect.

The theater group quickly announced its play and the visitors sat in a circle on the grass and waited with blank faces.

The play, performed by three adults in huge hats and attic clothes and several children in exaggerated and bizarre baby clothes, was about an old bad-tempered bear (in grey fur and eyebrows with shaking papier-mache claws) who stole the children's toys. At pretend night, the children went to sleep and the adults lay down and snored; then the bear shook and growled a-cross the clearing and snatched a doll or teddybear or toy train and galloped shaking back into hiding; the children awoke and cried and jumped up and down. This was repeated several times; then the adult players said, "We're going to get the toys back from that bear." They asked the children in the audience to help; all those from the group jumped up to join the adventure and a few of the visiting children. They got one toy back. This was repeated several times; each time more children joined. Finally the bear stood up and cried. Na explained that na loved toys. Na wept and danced a for-lorn dance and told the children that na never got any toys because na was too old. The children caucussed. Someone thought they should give the bear a toy or two. They argued and agreed; but whose? All said, Not mine! The bear grew angry and chased them. They ran home and then turned around and chased the bear, who ran home. They next decided that the bear could play with the toys for one hour each day if na was very good. They placed the toys in the center of the clearing and stood watch over the bear, who played with the toys a clumsy and exaggerated game that made

31

everyone laugh. While they laughed the bear tried to slip the train inside nan fur; they caught na and chased na away. Na begged that the hour wasn't over; with glee the children told na that na was bad. They relented and let na come the next day, when they watched more carefully and once again, na tried to stick the teddybear inside nan fur. The children were even angrier, but this time the bear didn't run, na stood and waved the teddybear high in the air. "This one is mine," na growled, and explained that the teddybear looked like na because it was made from a piece of nan own fur; na turned and stuck out nan rear and showed a huge tear in nan suit. The children were confused. "But I'll let you play with it one hour a day," the bear said. The children were divided. One of the visiting children said they should get the bear and kill na. Nicky agreed and shouted, "Come on! We'll skin na and make nan whole suit into teddybears for us to play with." The children chased the bear who ran outside the audience circle. In a few minutes the children returned with the bear suit.

"Come on right now." A visiting parent pulled nan child by the arm.

"I didn't get a piece of the bear," the child cried.

"Teddybears aren't made from real bears," the parent said.

"That wasn't a real bear and I want a piece of its fur." The child lay down and kicked.

The carpenter closed nan eyes as parent after parent dragged nan child off down the sidewalk. The young people started the songs. Visiting teenagers with tan surpriseless faces wandered over to listen.

Carter and Bert had set up their health booth by the driveway; their only concession to the carnival theme was a skeleton dangling from the jut of the booth, wearing a straw cartwheel hat covered with flowers and a tangerine chiffon scarf. They wanted to set up free health care and classes for the people of the community. They were handing out leaflets and talking to a few curious adults when the carpenter came near.

32

A visitor with eyes like pale seedless grapes was questioning Carter in a sharp voice. "Do you have any credentials? You have to have credentials to do a thing like that; after all, people want to know who you are before they're going to trust you."

"Credentials." Carter repeated the word as if na did not know its meaning. "Do you mean degrees, or experience?"

"Yes. Credentials."

"We have the experience of our own bodies." Carter was the only one of the group who still smiled; nan smile dislodged nan whole face and made it pop almost audibly at its target. The violence of the smile made Carter's simple sentence seem to mean something infinitely else. The visitor blinked and stepped back; Carter simultaneously leaned forward. "We all do. That's what I meant. You don't need a degree to fix a child's cut foot—you're better off without it because the degree would have told you to wash it in phisohex last year and not to wash it in phisohex this year. Our experience with lack of money would have told us to wash it in soap and water all along, just like our grandparents did. If it needs a stitch, you go to the hospital and we'll babysit for the other children."

"Oh well, if it's only cut feet . . ." The visitor was about to move away. "That's not so bad then." Nan disappointment expressed itself in nan first smile.

"It gets better," Carter said quickly. "We give all the usual tests—tuberculosis, diphtheria, pregnancy, diabetes, venereal disease, cervical cancer, lead poisoning, sickle-cell anemia . . ."

"Pregnancy?" The seedless grapes glistened as with a sudden spray.

"Sure. Free, for one thing, and no waiting."

"Well. I think you're in the wrong town. Our young people still get married, thank heavens." The voice recited this indignation as a matter of form; above, the eyes were green with curiosity. "You mean you examine people—girls—you give medical examinations and things like that?"

"We have classes to teach people how to examine themselves, too." Carter smiled deliberately, exaggerating naself. "Why, I bet you couldn't draw an accurate picture of female genitals with everything in the right place—clitoris, vagina, urethra, both sets of lips—they call them labia, you know . . ." Carter turned back, having found a pencil and paper but the visitor was gone.

"Well, here. You want to try?" Carter offered the pencil and paper to the carpenter.

While na was drawing, trying to remember ancient or recent scientific or pornographic pictures because, strangely enough, knowledge of such things comes almost entirely from books as if female genitals were in fact insides . . . a new visitor stood quietly by the edge of the booth reading a mimeographed health sheet. Nan eyes darted up at the carpenter drawing and Carter watching and back at the paper and up again. Carter saw na, saw nan mouth moving in minuscule tremors as if na were hungry and thinking about food, saw the twitches shiver into a broad grin when na caught Carter's eye.

Na identified naself as a resource redistributor and offered to help. Na was interested in health; na had never had any—"What couldn't I do with it since I make out pretty fair without it?" Na grinned again, "Am I allowed to smoke? I don't want to pollute the health booth. I didn't bring a bottle because I knew the law would like that and I try not to please the law too often, you know. One more time and they'll be pleased for good." Na blew smoke carefully toward the sidewalk. "I've been up twice already. Not bad, considering I've been working for twenty years. But once more will be it so I try to be careful now. I want to help you folks out though if I can. I'm a forger."

The carpenter held out nan picture for Carter to study.

"It certainly looks weird," the forger said.

34

"Is it right?" the carpenter said. "Does anybody know if it's right?"

"Meet a forger," Carter said, holding the drawing toward the light.

"Delighted. Really?"

"Resource redistributor." The forger held out a bony hand for the carpenter to shake. "I scoop a little off the top of the oil wells every year and spread it in the streets."

The carpenter held the hand as long as na dared. "Join us."

"Better not. If I was here the law'd be watching you folks like peeping Toms. I work best alone. Say, can I see that picture again?"

"Sure."

"Whatdya know. Certainly looks weird." Na handed it back and turned to find a spot to put out nan cigarette. "Hey. I know you," na said to the person no one had noticed, standing just off the booth—of huge height and build, na stood as square as an ox. "Yeah," the forger said, "I know you but I'm not introducing you to any friends of mine. What trouble are you looking for tonight?"

"Just curious to see the action." With a smile that reminded everyone of the reasons they had stopped smiling, the forger's acquaintance moved up to the booth and introduced naself. "Since Dallas here won't," na said. "They call me Tiny."

"Curious as a crocodile," Dallas said.

"Can I see your literature?" Tiny reached for the paper with the drawing on it; Carter intercepted the hand and filled it with mimeographed sheets most of which fell to the ground. "What are you hiding?" Tiny said then as the carpenter stuffed the drawing in nan back pocket. "You let that one look, now let me." Na thrust a bossy hand at the carpenter.

"That's my horoscope," the carpenter said.

"Sure it's not a map of buried treasure?" Na red-hot laugh was on top of the carpenter now.

The carpenter stood achingly still. "You know, for a light-head you sure come on heavy." Every anger in nan body tightened and longed to fight. Na concentrated nan will on urging this pale ox to hit or spit or push na. Dallas the forger had disappeared.

"I oughta ream you," Tiny hissed.

"You ought to leave while you're still rightside up," the carpenter said.

"Listen, you motherfucker . . . "

"You tell me, shitmouth."

From the edge of nan eye, the carpenter saw Carter standing equally tensed and ready by Tiny's side. Na did not see the others who had gathered just outside nan concentration. Na ached for the other to make the first move.

Tiny spat at the carpenter's face, missed, hit nan neck.

"Pissmouth. Sorry."

The carpenter saw the hand move back, moved nan own knee instantly up to Tiny's crotch, kicked as hard as na could. Tiny lost balance and fell. When na hit the ground, the carpenter sat on nan chest at the throat and held one arm, Carter simultaneously grabbed and held the other.

The cook ran out of the crowd and lunged for a foot, holding it down with nan weight; na was viciously kicked in the back with the other foot. Na tried to reach for it too and was kicked again on the arm.

"What the hell are you doing?" Stubby came slowly over.

"Grab the other foot," the carpenter said.

"What is going on here?" Stubby said.

The cook was kicked a third time, let go the leg na was holding and quickly got out of range. The freed legs strained in huge arcs, unbalancing the two holding the shoulders.

"For christsake, Stubby, hold nan legs!" the carpenter shouted.

"Oh, no you don't." Stubby tried to hold back two others who were ready to jump in for nan legs. Stubby circled with nan bulk in front of them as they tried to dodge past under nan arms.

One got through and grabbed a leg; it was Chris. At the same time the cook jumped back onto the other leg and sat, with a laugh of congratulations to Chris.

"We got the pig!" Chris shouted.

"What'd na do?" the cook asked.

Andy was crying because Stubby held na fast. "Let Andy go," Chris ordered but Stubby shook nan head. Na was explaining that violence was wrong and when we resort to violence we are just as bad as they are and besides, a victory won by violence is no . . .

Gulliver lay still and the captors' breathing returned to normal.

"What are we going to do with na?"

"We'll all have to let go at once."

"Where?"

Sitting on a person's flesh is a kind of intimacy. Carter's and the carpenter's hands were gripping their enemy's arms with an intensity and determination not to let go that one usually expends upon a most cherished person or (as a child) thing; they were both so close to nan face that they could count the eyebrow hairs, could look as deep into nan eyes as if na were a lover. The carpenter, who had so recently been that close with other emotions to the cook's flesh, felt the suction of attraction and revulsion, a magnetic confusion, on being thus on top of and interlocked with this enemy-stranger.

The body lay absolutely still but the eyes became compensatorily full of energy, seemed to be thrashing and hitting and aiming and thrusting with a physical force. Na was fucking them with nan eyes. Their choice was either to release that repulsive flesh and get far away, or smash it into the earth.

"Blindfold na," the carpenter said.

Nicky appeared with a piece of the bearsuit and tied it so tightly around the victim's eyes that nan mouth registered pain for the first time, and tried to bite

37

Nicky—opening to reveal yellow-stained, silver-filled teeth, and looking suddenly human.

Andy broke away from Stubby's grip and ran to the house, coming back with a length of rope. They tied the hands together then, in front because it was too risky to try to turn na over and move the hands to the back. They looped the rope between nan legs and back to nan waist, thus fastening the hands at the abdomen in front in a design like a g-string.

Na looked helpless and comical. Stubby turned nan back after telling them that they were animals and sick and no better than their attacker.

"What did na do?" the cook asked again.

"Get up," the carpenter said to the trussed figure, holding the waist rope firmly.

They pulled and pushed na to the sidewalk and headed na toward Main Street with a kick. "Someone will find na and then na can explain what happened . . . if na wants to," Carter said.

The carpenter turned with white rage in Stubby's direction and said from the sidewalk in a furious shout so all could hear, "You never, *never* HINDER someone in a fight! You might as well attack me yourself. I don't care *what* principles are involved."

Stubby called a meeting to discuss the disagreement.

Stubby spoke in nan own defense: "I've been through all this with the Marxists and the anti-McCarthyites and the Young Lords and the Panthers and the Jewish Defense League and I know one thing: if we use the same old methods we'll have the same old politics and deserve them. I don't care what that particular person did but I know I saw members of my own group handle the incident as if they were in a street fight. We have ways to handle such things—don't we have ways to handle such things? Haven't we spent meeting after meeting . . ."

"That's the trouble," the carpenter said.

"Don't interrupt . . ."

38

"Let na finish . . ."

"Yes, please; let me finish. It's you I'm talking to."

"Didn't you interrupt *me* and put Carter and me in danger of . . ."

". . . you, as I said. And I certainly know that you will answer what I say, have every right to answer— that's been decided too. To proceed now: in these meetings—which I happen to think are not a chore at all, but a chance to talk to each other and find out what everyone is thinking; a privilege, in fact—in these meetings we have repeatedly decided that *no one* is to handle a threat by naself, particularly the person who is emotionally involved . . ."

"Na irritates my soul to the seventh layer," the carpenter whispered to the cook.

"Because na knits," the cook whispered back. "Even when na talks, one row of words has one stitch, the next row a second and the whole thing is put together loop by loop and ends up looking solid. The only way you could tear down nan argument would be to pick it apart stitch by stitch, and you don't have small enough fingers to do that."

The carpenter kissed the cook's ragged fingernails. "You do."

"My trouble is that I agree with na," the cook said. "If only someone else were saying it."

"*It* would not be *it* if someone else were saying it."

"*It* is *it* only when we do it?"

"Shhhhh . . ."

". . . I also know that I'm going to be trashed for what I think, for going against spontaneity and courage and fighting back—as if we all adhered to the western saloon code of honor—but I want to make one further point: either I have an equal right to express my feelings as anyone else or the whole morality of this group is in question and that's all I want to say, that these are my honest feelings." Stubby's face had a rare look of almost-quiver, an unset expression which moved over nan solid features as if tickled from below by what na

39

claimed: honest feeling.

"As for feeling," the carpenter said in the waiting silence. "I was scared."

"Yeah," Carter said.

"There's the story of the aristocrat," the carpenter said. "Who was carefully taught to walk with a graceful and delicate step. One spring na was out in the woods shooting spotted ponies because na wanted to panel the walls of nan bedroom in spotted ponyskin. 'Panel' is is wrong but 'paper' would be worse. Na took aim and shot nan third pony, but when na went to retrive the skin na saw that it was not a pony at all but a person whose heavy step had confused the aristocratic ear trained to soundlessness. Now is the point of this story that the aristocrat can't even tell the difference between nan own kind and an animal?" No one knew what the point of the story was, but the carpenter waited nevertheless for some kind of answer.

Stubby offered it. "The last thing I ever thought anyone could accuse me of is being an aristocrat." Nan stubborn body stood firm in outrage and envy. "Weaving is not the same thing as shooting ponies for their skins." Instantly everyone saw the rugs and macrame hangings, which crowded the walls of Stubby's room so closely that they covered like wallpaper, as an unusual kind of aristocracy but nevertheless spotted somehow with perversion.

The carpenter's rage slipped soundlessly away.

4

The cook's hair smelled of cigarette smoke and charcoal and faint hamburger; the carpenter breathed the combination into nan brain to quiet the one anger that na could not speak about and did not want to think about: na first disappointment with the cook's way of making love. The gentleness of nan touch, now, after less than a week, irritated the carpenter; the hand sliding over nan head and back was so parentally soothing, so tender and loving, that the carpenter thought na would burst from hidden tears of grief. The slight scratching of the cook's ragged fingernails, the one-time accidental yank of the carpenter's pubic hair, an occasional pressure into pain on nan genitals themselves, were all apologized for with such tender strokes of love that the carpenter felt all desire slink away.

Na smelled again for the smoke and charcoal and carnival meal and lay wrapped in the cook's arms as

41

quietly as creamed chicken in a pancake. The carpenter's initial desire, arising each night and each hour they were together in the night, lunged toward the cook with the intensity of an unknown poem and culminated in more than satisfaction, in something the carpenter had never before experienced—a total human orgasm. A second voice challenged the first voice's greed: then what more? A third defended the first's need to speak: I do want more; sometimes I want to lie soft as water waiting for the cook's hands to set me into involuntary movement, to lie innocent as a child . . . but what happens then is that the cook caresses me like silk, as if na were bathing an infant and smoothing it with oil.

The carpenter took a gulp of smell to dilute nan arms' urge to squeeze nan lover until na cried. Unless I respond, na thought, the cook can't act. Na is too sensitive; na has spent nan life feeling what other people— the other person—feel(s); it is the instinct of the short and the method of the timid. Na never creates a situation of nan own. And so the other . . . and so *I* never get the excitement of being suddenly pulled into another's world.

"Hey," cried the cook in the voice of *ouch*. "What are you doing?"

"I'm sorry. I didn't mean to hurt you." The carpenter loosened nan arms' grip, sat free and looked at the cook's face.

Moving soft and infinitesimal like a flower growing in and out of itself, the beauty of that face caught at the carpenter's chest like the clutch of a baby's hand and all thoughts of the offensive infant oil were reabsorbed in that moment's touch. "Your face," na said, staring at that life six inches away. "Your face . . ." Nan hand barely touched a cheek's incurve. Na stared, paralyzed by the sudden fact that the face na loved was alive and six inches away. Fear swooped down over nan consciousness like a predatory shadow. "Talk to me," na cried, closing off that face by digging nan own into the flat side of the cook's shoulder. "Talk to me," na said again in a swallowed whisper.

The cook's practiced hand stroked nan back in soothing circles and nan other arm held the carpenter's head like a cradle.

5

In most groups there are whispers, a term that has little to do with the volume of the speaking voice but refers rather to the peregrinations of what is said: phrases wander from ear to mouth to ear, during a walk across grass, down a hall to work, behind a door in the bathroom, at varying distances from the people or events which are their subject, leaving a trail of uneasy excitement throughout the routine. Words are passed along like hasty pats, the person speaking making no more serious commitment to them than the recipient, sometimes with a laugh, sometimes with a future-aimed frown, always with the meaning though that we should wait and see.

By the time the carpenter ran across the trail, several verbal days had gone by.

Na was working in the garage, making two bookcases for money. Na had also agreed to remodel a garage into a studio for money. Na was singing a half-voiced, half-mouthed song on the first October day that was slightly cool—seventy-two—a break in the temperature of summer which whispered that the heat was essentially over. But the carpenter was really listening to the whispers of the wood by which a board suggested that it be laid this way not that. Na stood now stroking with nan eye the incredible curves of the grain. The time before beginning to make any structure, the minutes after the wood is in front of you but before you take any tool to it, was to the carpenter a period of pure happiness and nan body felt sprung from the earth like a tree itself in joy.

Therefore na was angry that someone should choose those minutes to intrude the trail of the whispers, and the anger produced a useful deafness.

"Stubby is leaving," the one called Tracy said, the one who drove a taxi for a local fleet but who was only really interested in writing. Because na wrote, na wandered around the group when na was not working, trying to find out who everyone was. Na had not gotten to the carpenter before.

The carpenter said, "Good." Na had misunderstood.

Stubby was not going to leave just like that. Na had told everyone including people who shared the group's politics in Chicago, Boston, New York and Berkeley. Na had written a statement, detailing nan position and enemies, and intended to read it tonight at a meeting. Na had sent a copy of the statement to Chicago, Boston, New York and Berkeley.

There were two main charges in the statement: that Stubby was being treated as if na were a pig and that personal dislike of na was infiltrating the movement.

That night they got word that one called Three was coming down to pay their group a visit. From Chicago. A change came over everyone; their faces showed that they were straightening out their politics as if they were cleaning up the house for a visitor.

45

It was very unreal.

"Na is leaving because of you," the cook said. A large number of the whispers had passed by the stove and across the chopping table. "Everybody knows that you don't like Stubby—after Saturday night no one could miss knowing it. And you have a lot of influence here."

"I don't want that kind of influence—to be 'followed.'" The carpenter had once wanted that, and even now experienced as a kiss the cook's admiration when na spoke of nan lover's influence. But the chill followed so fast that the kiss was cold before it reached the brain: the carpenter knew that to be followed was the prerequisite for being dumped and na wanted more than anything to belong.

"What you say is important to people, that's all. There's nothing you can do about it. People have learned to value your mind because it is clearer than most of ours, and usually fair. So then the rare time it is not completely fair . . . those who don't know you all that well value what you say then too."

"I'm going to have to be perfect, then."

"You could apologize."

"Godammit, everybody gets to say what na is feeling except me. I have to hold everything in until I'm sure I'm not just reacting emotionally to my own hangups—no one else had to do this, just me. I have to be a goddamn holy parent. An editor. A spokesperson for the movement. Stubby had more time than I did to tell everyone how wrong I was."

"Stubby needed even more time. Na doesn't understand naself or you well enough to explain how na was right. And besides," the cook grinned, "na has that irritating way of saying anything."

The carpenter was sitting in the center of an energy field of anger and stood up, sat down, stood up, turned and turned back. The cook could light a cigarette but the carpenter would not; na forced nan brain to carry the anger until it exploded.

"I have marvelous choices," na said, the words pushing each other out very fast and clear. "I can apologize to Stubby and whoever else wants to listen—I can say that I am clearer-headed than na is and should not take advantage of this gift of mine; I should instead grow muddled to give na a fair chance. If I force myself to grow muddled, na might feel that I am the patronizing parent crawling on the floor with the children. If I remain silent to allow Stubby plenty more time to say what na needs so much time to say, the whole group may feel that they are getting to hear only one person and then doesn't Stubby become the one with too much influence? If I scream and complain about na in private, to you, to let off steam so I can be cool in the meetings, I am being private and talking about people behind their backs not to their faces. However, if I tell na exactly what I think of na, everyone else might be influenced to get rid of na absolutely. Stubby naself might be crushed beyond the repair of those most dedicated to we-have-to-support-each-other. So if it's impossible for both of us to co-exist in one group, one of us will have to leave, and it'll be me since I'm the one who cares too much about the group to let it collapse beneath Stubby's and my mutual antagonisms. And that's always the way—the group loses the one person who is most dedicated to it. I'm going to go out and get drunk."

Paralyzed from habit, from the past when na was impotent to stop the child who screamed and ran away, the lover who raged and slammed the door, the parent who cursed and drank and stayed away, the cook sat stone still and trembling while the carpenter moved toward the door, checking nan pockets for money and keys. Na was not moving fast, the cook saw. "Wait," the cook said, barely audibly.

"Wait." The cook took nan arm, nan shoulder, held nan face with nan own. "I love you. Don't go."

For a moment the carpenter's body began to cry, hold me, hold on, hold, hold. But na abruptly let go and stepped back. Na was furious, too angry to feel the love that nan mind said was there. "I can't stay here and rave at you. That's no help and unfair to you. I'm going out to get drunk." Na did not move toward the door, however. "Why can't Stubby just go— leave, storm out, walk out, run away, stamp nan feet, slam the door and be done with it! Godammit, na leaves but na won't leave. We're going to be tied up in nan leaving for days and then na'll stay so na can leave again next week. I should have let na handle that belligerent one they call Tiny all by naself and let na get the shit beaten out of na and then na could leave because no one stepped in to help na."

The cook said quickly, "You didn't hate na before that night though. I did."

"You're smarter than *I* am."

"I never felt I had to like na in the first place. Na was here and I accepted that, but I didn't think I had to like na too. But you did. You spent all that time understanding the point na might have had. It's like what the moon said to the dough: you're not doing anything but rising, you just look different when you do it."

The carpenter's frown slipped away and nan voice which had been flat as tin, softened. "Okay, you're a fucking poet, you are."

"Come here." The cook reached out and held the carpenter urgently close. "You are my child, my own precious child, come here and let me hold you."

"I'm here," the carpenter murmured through a mesh of hair.

"Now I'm going to get you something to eat," the carpenter said after a timeless period of time, an acting love that had swamped and filled them both coming as it did onto their already spinning emotions—the carpenter's rage and the cook's fright that na would not be quick enough to turn the

rage around. "I'm going to feed the world's feeder. Then you can tell me the best thing to do, the
choice I haven't thought of."

"I'll tell you a story," the cook said, before
starting the second half of nan sandwich but keeping the beer nevertheless resting close on nan knee,
because it was a surprise. "I thought I knew everything that was anywhere in that refrigerator. I didn't
know we had beer. You know Stubby has gotten
to know a lot of people who have power in this
town, because na speaks Spanish and works in the
Center and likes to talk politics. Na thinks that
if we're careful—if we let Stubby do our talking—
that the people who run this town can be won
over to support us, or at least to accept the fact
that we're here. Na said yesterday that it looks like
they want a favor from us in return, if we took in a
certain number of homeless people and children and
helped obliterate that blot on their town's shining
surface. Stubby said, 'If we run a refuge for blots.' "

The carpenter laughed out loud. "Good. I didn't
know na had a sense of humor."

"That's arrogant, too, of course—to accept na
for that."

"I'm arrogant. It's also using na, to accept na
for a front."

"What choice do we have?"

"Or maybe it's not. The two things we are trying to do—set up a counterculture and make a
revolution . . . it's hard to do both things at the
same time. So people like Stubby who are devoting
all their energies to one thing, who aren't sidetracked
by looking for personal happiness—we need people
like that. And it's easier for Stubby too in a way,
since na is only interested in the revolution part."

"Easier? But na also has no personal world.. . ."

"Simpler."

". . . to live in, no sustenance or comfort. Na is

not in love and doesn't even have friends na loves. We should be able to understand how lonely na must feel, how left out and jealous of those who are in love. Darling, we should feel sorry for the rest of the world."

"Na is in love with you! Fuck it, I'm sure of it."

"Na isn't."

"Of course na is. Everyone is." The carpenter stood up and towered above the cook, who was sitting cross-legged like a child on the bed. "This whole display is for you—writing letters and making speeches and calling meetings and getting that person down here from Chicago . . . Three. Na is creating a storm to get your attention, to force you to choose nan side, to make you notice na and see how much na loves you and to what great lengths na would go for you."

"That's really unfair. You're saying nan politics is motivated by that old desire to win love and approval and that's all."

"Wait a minute." The carpenter sat back down. "That is what I'm saying . . . let me think a minute. Aha! I know. Look, I really don't believe that anyone can work for a revolution separate and distinct from nan own personal happiness or love-needs. Such a person wouldn't have any way of knowing the difference between what is true and what false. It isn't that we're trying to do two things at once—set up a counterlife and work for a revolution; the two are halves of the same whole and the absolutely essential thing is to keep juggling them. If we concentrate on either one and forget the other we produce a monster. That's Stubby's definition; na is a monster and nothing na says, even when na is 'right,' is really right."

"Stubby is not a monster," the cook said firmly.

"You don't understand what I mean by monster. I mean na does everything by thinking and analyzing and reasoning, and na doesn't pay attention to who na is and what na is feeling. I think that *is* a monster. Or becomes or produces or might as well be a monster."

"You don't mean the term as an insult . . . but it *is*."

50

"So then it is. I'm going to get us another beer."

"I have to go to sleep. It's very late."

"Do you?"

"I have to get up early."

"You do. I'll go back to my room."

"How can you?"

"You're right. I can't." The carpenter crawled into the mattress on the floor and lay close to the cook. "I'll sleep here with you, crowded and beerless." Na put nan arm under the cook's shoulders and held na close. "Because we love each other. Don't we?"

Why despair? The carpenter moved gently away from the cook's sleeping arm curved across nan lover's back, stopped still when the cook tightened nan grip on the carpenter's hand, waited until the grip loosened and then slipped the hand away, leaving the cook's hand to reach in sleep and settle finally into a fist pushed under nan own belly. The carpenter stood by the window, breathing deeply, quickly awake with the feeling that na had escaped. At once na sat back down on the mattress on the floor and put nan hand lightly on the cook's extended leg, loving na through that symbolic touch and ashamed na had thought, escape.

But why despair? The carpenter's whole mind and body longed for another beer, na total consciousness was irritable and diffused and craved alcohol to drop nan mind into its patterns or apparent patterns which served the same purpose as real ones could have done. After several minutes spent talking naself into and out of the trip to the kitchen, na decided that the argument was the real waste of time and went to the kitchen for another beer.

The trip, the new room empty and dark, the different light through different windows, caught nan imagination and fed it briefly with visual patterns; then na sat at the kitchen table with nan beer and asked again, why despair?

The burden the cook is putting on me—of being

51

strong—is throwing me back into that intolerable position again: parent. Na tells me I am strong so na can sleep easily wrapped in the knowledge that na has told me. Na even tells me I am so strong I don't need to go out and drink myself out from under the burden and leaves me awake and ashamed of myself for now unjustifiably doing just that.

Clarity came with the last swallow of this beer hastily drunk. Since I weaken my reason with drink, I can no longer be expected to understand that I am too strong to need to drink.

The next beer na took to the back porch and the carpenter sat on its edge in the moonlight thinking about nan own edge.

In alcoholic catalogue, na found naself listing the reasons for joy; most of them concerned the cook and that love found. But the more na listed, the longer the list, the more it became clear that, like a devious taxpayer's return, the same thing was being counted many times: the cook, one person, one love, was in truth only one joy. The carpenter was forced to concede to the nagging feeling of despair that other platitude: the same food which can drive a person to obsessive lengths to obtain is, once eaten, accepted by the mind as well as the belly and little thought of. Now what? despair wanted to know and the question rang with the undertone of, so what?

So the questions were back, the questions na had thought forever past had only been on a little trip, away less than a month and full of renewed health and vigor after their vacation. To attack now in the moonlight a mind gentle with beer. Na thought of gin: the sharp bite of that stronger cold whiteness could speed nan mind to deal with the questions in five minutes and then obliterate them. There was one hotel where na might be able to buy gin at this hour, for a huge cost both in money and to nan own mind now open and soft. Na finished the beer and went inside for another, but na knew that nan stomach could not hold enough of its volume to benefit from its minor alcohol.

Na took this beer across the moonlit backyard which stretched back an eighth of a mile, to a large willow whose tears reached to the ground. Inside that umbrella, na curled nan back into the angle where the trunk met the earth. Na gripped the beer can which bent easily; it was as weak and temporary as its contents.

I held and adored my lover earlier this same night and now I feel nothing of love; verbal memory only remains. I know that I love na but I feel nothing. I know that I have never loved anyone as much as I love the cook but I feel nothing. I only know love from my own loving, which tells me that loving someone completely more than anything ever on earth means sometimes feeling nothing, not one ounce of love for na. Feeling nothing but remembering that one did feel two hours ago is to feel something after all—the pain of the difference between the two.

My bones are dissolving, the frame which supports my flesh is melting and I will soon be the shape of dumped wet cement which will harden uselessly. My teeth are clenched and my mouth contracted and there is no room for food inside it at all. My eyes are open to no purpose except that when they close the darkness is confusion pounding dark against my eyelids. I am curled into the past because it is only there that I can breathe so shallowly that consciousness fades, because the past is so far back because I am so old, too old, much too old to dare to go wake the cook and shout, how dare you go to sleep and leave me old and dareless?

The carpenter woke the next morning as the first light came through the glistening green of the willow threads. Na neck was stiff and would not turn and na knees ached like a tired child's. Na laid naself on the grass and wept, nan mind furry and vulnerable. The greatest love na had ever known was not enough.

6

By ten o'clock the carpenter had cut two boards wrong: once because na had not allowed for the top board of the bookcase to be two board thicknesses longer than the inside boards, the second time because na had cut along a pencil line made for an inside board before the board had been chosen for the top because of its more graceful grain. Nan mind was preoccupied with its own lack of sleep. Guilt from the hangover was punishing nan pocketbook sternly.

Outside the garage Andy and Chris stopped laughing as na approached.

"What's so funny?" the carpenter said.

"Last night . . ." Andy started laughing again.

"You see, last night . . ." Chris could barely keep from laughing too. "We were both stoned and Andy . . . Andy sat down on a parked car. But the trouble was, there wasn't any car there." The laugh broke loose.

"We both saw the car but when Andy sat down, na was in the street."

"I busted my ass," Andy said and laughed. "It wasn't funny; it hurt."

"It wasn't funny but it was," Chris said. "We couldn't stop laughing. That car was there and Andy sat down on it and it wasn't there. It was so funny." Chris laughed again. "If you could have seen Andy's face when the car turned into the pavement!"

"I was on my ass in the street where the car was and we couldn't stop laughing," Andy said. "I still can't."

"Then I said, 'I'll prove to you the car isn't there,' " Chris said. "And I sat down on the car and landed on the pavement too!"

The carpenter felt laughter coming up from nan own belly. Then they heard the shouts of the children from the side yard.

"I am a tiger!" a boy cried.

"I am a lion!" a second boy said.

"I'm a fox," a third boy said.

"I'm an eagle!" a girl's voice shouted.

"Goose!" a boy threw back.

"Gander!" the girl said.

"Goose. Goose. Goose. Goosie, goosie, goose," the third boy repeated.

"Gander. Rooster!" a second girl shouted.

"Hen!"

"Biddy!"

"Chick, chick, chick!"

"Ox! Dumb ox!"

"Cow!"

"Sow!"

"Bull!"

"Yeah, I'm a bull! Cow, sow, cow, sow, hen, cat!"

"Dog!"

"Butterfly!"

"Magpie!"

"Chickadee!"

"Crow! Old crow!"

55

"Old goat!"

"Hog! hog! hog, hog! Ox, hog, dog, goat!"

"Lamb, filly, kitten, dove, pigeon, piglet!"

"Ant!"

"Snake!"

"Worm!"

"Skunk!"

"Bitch!"

"Bitch!"

"Shrimp!"

"Ant!"

"Shark!"

"Hawk!"

"Tomcat!"

"Pussy!"

"Pussy!"

"Cock!"

"Pussy! pussy! pussy! pussy! pussy!"

"Hog, dog, ox, snake, worm, skunk, shrimp!"

The small female voice grew weaker and shriller; the small male voices boomed like those of ordained men.

"Bitch!"

"Pussy!"

"Ass!"

"Pussy!"

"Cock!"

"Pussy!"

"Bitch!"

"Ass!"

"Cow!"

"Cow!"

"Cow!"

"Shut up! SHUT UP, SHUT UP, SHUT UP!" The carpenter shouted and lunged for the children, nan face clenched with rage and nan arms waving and threatening as na chased the nearest children. "You goddamn phony two-bit little . . . little . . . you're nothing but a *kid*!" na screamed, catching one, the cook's squirming, kicking youngest.

"You're nothing but a goddamn *kid*!" The carpenter slapped the child across the bottom and pushed na away. The carpenter's head pounded and nan arm ached to beat all of them at once until nan head was blind. "Get out of here!"

Chris called nan name softly as the carpenter passed. From the side the carpenter saw nan face, troubled and young with the urge to help, but the carpenter kept nan own eyes furiously away.

"It's their obscenity. That's all. It's . . ."

The carpenter pulled down the garage door, deafening naself with a loud long rattle of metal and parts.

7

Three arrived the following Friday afternoon, in a Volkswagen bus with a companion from Chicago and people they had picked up in St. Louis and Little Rock . . . seven in all, they brought produce and bedrolls and three recorders and squatted on the group playing, "Deep in the Heart of Texas." A local bakery truck pulled into the driveway behind them. Its driver unloaded three boxes of bread and sweet rolls and immediately drove off.

"Who was that?"

"Look!"

"A friend who wants to help us," Three said. "We found na at a traffic light."

The cook met the boxes of bread and sacks of produce with the pure smile feeders reserve for groceries. Then na saw Three. "Pete!" the cook cried. "You're . . . ?"

"It's me." Three dumped the box of bread and

grinned at the cook.

"What a surprise," the cook said. "I mean, I am surprised but I should know better than to be surprised by anything you do. I had no idea . . . you're Three? When did you do that? It doesn't matter . . ." Na stopped, seeing the question in Three's eyes. They hadn't seen each other since the year of the cook's divorce—two years ago; the cook searched back for nan politics of that year. Na remembered. Na pulled back, prepared to defend nan changes.

"This is Scott," Three said.

"Hi."

"Sure."

"And Teddy and Norton and Jojo and Sidney and Val. You look different. Good. New? I can't talk when there's food around."

"I remember," the cook said.

"We'll fix dinner," Scott said.

The carpenter had taken the cook's children on a supper picnic down to the bayou, to look for snakes. A guilt trip. They would not be back until after dinner; the cook had two hours before the carpenter would meet Three; nevertheless na was uneasy.

The cook sat on the grass with a huge sack of beans. Three had taken off na shirt and was lying in the late sun. Na eyes were half-closed. The cook avoided them as if they had been wide open; Three's eyes had a way of watching when you spoke which made you feel that you were lying even when you weren't. Or didn't know you were. Or hadn't meant to. Or . . .

Na snapped the beans as if na would play a tune on the first musical instrument invented by cooks. They could talk about food: Three's feet had been dirty all nan life and nan belly afraid—although it was almost never empty now, fear hung around the edges of every delayed meal. Each movement march or demonstration which took na away from a kitchen for long hours would find Three with one eye always on the path of the hot dog carts. The habit of fearing hunger was such that the kitchen was the only place indoors where na could feel easy. The cook snapped off the stem of a bean and dropped it into Three's mouth.

"Tell me what's going on down here," Three said.

The cook told na about the threat of attack the egg-woman brought, the carnival, the fight between Stubby and the carpenter and where they were now.

"So you're in love with the carpenter," Three said when the cook had finished.

"What does that mean anymore?"

"Are you?"

"In-love is that feeling kids get when they go to the movies and look in the mirror a lot." The cook threw Three another bean and ate one naself.

Three laughed. "I thought I was the cynic, but even I don't believe that."

"It's just insane to have four children," the cook said softly, looking at the beans. "And I'm not ready to make it alone. I thought I was, when I got the divorce, but that was really you. Because you were strong I borrowed from you and when you were around I stopped distinguishing what was borrowed and what was really me. You gave me that—courage to try alone. But that was then."

"You don't have to do it alone," Three said.

"I'm the only one of the group who doesn't contribute any money at all. That's why I do the cooking. And I have the worst kid. The carpenter . . . I need someone to help me." The cook put the beans aside and waited for Three to say something. Na didn't. The cook spent a long time searching nan pockets for a cigarette and match, lit a cigarette, and continued in a voice nervous with defiance: "Nicky was thrown out of school last week and school only started three weeks ago. I knew na would be. Na stole and wrote insults on the blackboards and all over the toilets. The assistant principal called na in and Nicky threw a tantrum and started tearing up the office. Then na ran home. I went

60

to see the principal but they don't want na back and I don't blame them. The truant officer'll be next. And then the group will throw us out. They'll say it's because it isn't right for one person to be the cook, everyone should share and all that, but it'll be because of Nicky. It always is."

"Where's Nicky now?"

"The carpenter took na to look for snakes because the carpenter lost nan temper with the little one over something Nicky started but no one can catch Nicky. The snake won't get na either. Besides they took along a snake-bite kit."

"You know I really dig that kid."

"Yeah. Other people do."

"So if Nicky wasn't around you'd be in love with the carpenter, or could . . ."

"Oh, Jesus Christ," the cook said and then laughed. "Sure I would. And I'd be nineteen and my hair would be black and when I sat down my stomach wouldn't roll over my jeans. I'd be in love and I'd dance on the streets and I'd feel sorry for those people with children but not very sorry because I'd know that I was special, I would do it differently, I'd never get caught in that trap. And my eyes would be clear: I'd look at Stubby and see that na works and has a program for getting the town on our side and since I wouldn't care whether the town was on our side or not I'd call it compromise (meaning shit) and decide with my own fresh free mind that Stubby couldn't be trusted because na isn't in love."

"Now you know I didn't have children because I didn't want to do what I had to do to get them, that's all. I didn't want to love or live with or have anything to do with those others. I sure never thought I was out-thinking you or anyone else."

Nevertheless Three lay lean and tanned in the afternoon sun, with only a small, single, unwrinkled pad of flesh above nan belt and hair consistently brown; the cook felt thought-out. Three was thirty-seven.

61

"People with kids can't be revolutionaries unless they're really forced to it," the cook said. "We'll always compromise if we can."

"I know," Three said, and the resonance and depth that came up through that flat Virginia accent cracked the cook's defensive wall. "We all compromise. Don't you know that? We get scared or hungry or our needs are too much for us. But we don't have to make compromise our philosophy."

"Do it, just don't admit it."

"Admit it but don't make a fucking program out of it." Three sat up and put nan hand on the cook's knee. Nan eyes were brown and direct and too intense; the cook felt their power as an electrical current tickling and soothing nan mind. The tension left and na sat very still. Na tried to listen.

"When you feel you are stuck in an oppressive relationship, for whatever reason, you learn to justify and defend it even if it is necessary to restructure the consciousness and rearrange everything you know. No, listen to me; we all do this. We begin to reach philosophical conclusions from personal needs. And we even say, that's what our movement is about: the personal is political. But the philosophy is supposed to come from the experience of our personal self, which is very different from dragging it in to justify a need. Take the scientists who try to prove that male animals are dominant because male humans feel insecure and need power, as opposed to the scientists who say, I and other male humans feel insecure; why? It's important to call a need a need. And then together we can remember or learn or imagine ways to satisfy it or, in some cases, like cannibalism, de-tooth it. And people who are in love are closer to calling a need a need than those who mainly think. It's only in that sense that I would distrust Stubby myself—I don't know where na is starting from."

"And me."

"I know where you're starting from," Three said. "I

was there."

"Underwater. I'm trying to learn to breathe underwater because I need to breathe. If I could fall in love, I guess I could burst through the surface into air and breathe easily. Then why don't I?"

"Maybe someone you care about is underwater with you."

"Maybe someone is holding me under and laughing maniacally," the cook said. "If we're talking about Nicky that seems more likely."

"That's why I'm here." Three stood up and stretched and grinned at the last red ball of sun. "I really came down hoping the Trots were trying to take over. I'd dig throwing them out. But look," na put a hand lightly on the cook's shoulder. "If they throw kids out of their schools we'll start our own schools. We're going to have to anyway."

"We saw a magnificent king snake." The carpenter slipped in to sit beside the cook. Na whispered because the meeting had already begun. "And Nicky caught a black widow spider."

The cook shivered.

Three's flat southern twang pricked at the carpenter's memory. Na spoke rapidly and clearly, although just noticeably louder than usual, with the excitement of a newcomer and a guest.

". . . whole thing seems to have gone off sideways from the start. You can't meet an enemy with a carnival and expect to be taken seriously. You've got real enemies here; we all do—outside and inside. Outside is easy. They're our enemies because we're a real threat to them and we can't sidestep that by pretending we're just into carnivals and games. We're serious and we know it. That's a middle-class university idea, to have a party. We'll have a party after the revolution, plenty of them. But now we have to talk to the people of this town and let them know we're dead serious."

The carpenter had read Three's writings, heard nan

63

voice once at a large meeting where na had been too far away to see Three and had only heard nan voice strike like a southern fist. But mainly the carpenter knew Three by what others said: whether political allies or enemies, everyone spoke of Three in a way to make one expect a huge, harsh, bull-person, not this compact purring southerner.

Three was physically perfect for a revolutionary. There was not an excess marble of fat on nan body. Na was the street cat not the lion—lean, muscular, of a smaller size the better to dart unnoticed through city life without calling attention to naself. Nan face was gentle, nan eyes in particular open and fresh and unafraid to face yours as long as you would. Coupled with the southern voice, Three's physical presence was captivating rather than ominous and the carpenter was having trouble matching the actual Three to the reputation.

"Now I don't want to add to the heat and forget about the light," Three said. "What happened at the carnival between two of you is important, partly because it happens in every group. The first thing to know is whether any internal disruption is the work of an agent for someone else or whether it is really an organic disagreement to be worked out. I'm for looking first for the agent because I know they're here and everywhere. But nobody else agrees with me, so we'll pass on that."

The carpenter was absorbed in watching Three's round brown eyes sparkle and dart into every face present and nan body arch and plead in a way that was both seductive and guerrilla-challenging. Three spoke as if na were anyone off the street who had come in to help; yet nan words sent a chill up the flesh of the carpenter for that very reason.

The chill changed to a tickle and made na sneeze. Three turned and grinned. The carpenter was aware of feeling what na had been unconsciously experiencing ever since Three started to talk; an electric attraction for Three which was sensual, genital and mental. Mental was strongest but the word doesn't convey—what the carpenter was feeling was nan mind and Three's connected, swooping, pulsating, jabbing together as possibility, as reality. Three's words and presence were beginning to excite the fantasy wheel of the carpenter's imagination. The carpenter was paralyzed, there against the wall as the politics were argued.

"Now if there's not an agent—I hope there is so I can find na—then we're up against our own violence and fear. It's no good to say, 'I'm against violence;' we're all violent somewhere underneath because we were raised in a violent society and we were the victims. Some of us want to be violent back every chance we get and others are too afraid from having been hit too much—they just want to get away. But nobody in this movement has really worked it out, that I've seen. So the first thing we ought to do is start having consciousness-raising on violence. How do we really feel about it? And I know one thing, the safe middle-class people may not think it applies to them but the working class *knows*. We've lived with violence since we were born and it's real all right. I know because I come from a place most of you read about in the magazines. So maybe we can teach our middle-class friends something for a change. If they want to listen, that is. We wouldn't want to *force* them to listen."

After a moment's silence, Chris said, "I really resent you coming in to tell us what to think or even, especially, what we are thinking."

Stubby said quickly, "You can't resent Three when na is going to all this trouble trying to help us."

"But I do."

"Well, you shouldn't," Stubby said.

"I still do." Chris laughed slightly to cover nan embarrassment, nan face flushed.

"Yeah, but wait a minute," Leslie said. Leslie was sitting next to Chris and the carpenter saw it suddenly: Leslie and Chris. "What you just said about the violence bit is right on. I know it's inside me. It's been there for as long as I can remember. And if it takes somebody from outside to come down here and put us back on our feet or back on our ass or wherever we're supposed to be . . . well, that's better than us going to hind part before and pretending it isn't so."

"It's the tone of it," Chris said. "Like we're not capable of working things out for ourselves. Even if we fuck up I'd like to . . ."

"Maybe we're not," Leslie said.

"Why did you come?" Tracy said. "I gather this isn't just a friendly visit?"

"Did anyone tell you to come?" Carter said.

Three said, "I . . ."

Stubby stood up. "I did. I want to read you the letter I wrote and sent out . . ."

"We all know what's in the letter," the carpenter said. "Just say what you want to."

"I want to read it." Stubby began reading.

"If you read it later, you could talk to us now, while you're feeling something you want to say. To us. If you read it now, you'll think you've said it all, but the letter will take the place of your talking directly to us, your pals all except me. And I'll shut up."

Stubby began reading. The letter was long and tediously phrased, latinate words all.

Carter interrupted. "Forget the letter, Stubby. Why did you get Three down here and lead na to think na was supposed to advise us?"

"Let na finish."

"Yeah."

Stubby finished the sentence na was reading. "That's why. 'Individuals must be made to realize that groups like ours are not autonomous or isolated bodies but are extremely important factors of the social struggles of all oppressed people that are manifesting themselves in the nation today.' Unless we unite behind socialism we will remain a club of friends talking over personal problems and not changing anything. It is imperative that we learn group and self-discipline. And I happen to know that Three is both disciplined and dedicated and that we need the perspective of someone from outside like na. Otherwise we'll fail." Stubby's voice cracked on "fail" and the tremor in nan face as na sat down showed that this was the worst thing that could happen to na, to fail.

There was murmuring throughout the room but no one spoke. Three said finally, "I'm not going to talk but once more. We really did come down because we wanted to take a trip, but we thought we had to offer some advice or such shit to . . . we understood that's what you wanted, all of you. So now we're going to be just friends visiting. I think the person who said . . . you in the black vest," na indicated Chris . . . "is right; I'd sure resent me if I was you. I'm glad you said it. And I think you're all beautiful because, well, look—a club of friends can be a powerful weapon." Na ducked behind nan companion and hugged na.

"We *saw* a king snake. We didn't catch one." The carpenter had caught up. Three was Pete, the cook's old friend. They were sitting at a table in the neighborhood bar. Three had sat down next to the cook, then had moved to the carpenter's end of the table. Now nan chair hung at a corner between the carpenter and Tracy. The cook was on a long diagonal. Stubby was absent.

The carpenter got up to get another beer, brushing Three's arm. It was as hard as nan own.

"You're right about the carnival. It was frivolous." The carpenter distributed nine beers, proud of nan own efficient fingers which so easily carried so many. "That was one reason we attacked that one called Tiny. We didn't really know that na had come just to . . . that na was part of a plan like the egg-woman said. We were predisposed to fight, our adrenalin was raging, and having a carnival took that away . . . from some of us." The carpenter found naself uneasily close to claiming superior knowledge from the start. "We sure could have

67

used you," na said with a laugh.

"The middle class can always use the working class on the front lines," Three said.

"Put it that way if you have to." The carpenter's voice trembled with anger.

Three grinned. "I knew the minute you opened your mouth that you came from the rich. It's written all over you. Those bones are too straight for us and you don't move like you learned how in the fields. But that voice clinches it: the way words that nobody else dares use slide out so naturally. You've got that soft slow southern overcoat on your words that sure dresses them up and you didn't learn that on tobacco road. I just wanted the pleasure of checking myself out, that's all."

"It's your pleasure."

"I'm selfish sometimes. But you're cool." Three leaned close, nan arm against the carpenter's. "It's just that I don't trust the rich. Sometimes I like them, I admire them and I sure do envy them. I just don't trust them. But we don't need to trust each other anyway, do we?"

The carpenter didn't answer.

"Look, I like you," Three said. "You're my old buddy's lover. You're smart. It's just that I come from where we learned to fight so young that when we get old we mix it up just for fun. Now I've ruined everything." Three laughed loudly to include the whole table. "I've been fighting so long its addled my wits. I can't carry on a decent conversation any more. Somebody help me." Na turned to Chris. "You in the black vest. What can I say now?"

"You stay away from my child," the carpenter said.

Back in nan own room, the carpenter poured warm gin from a pint bottle into a paper cup and knew na was very drunk. Patrician face said to mirror: I know I don't look like a drunk. Na took off clothes and swayed for naself and mirror. Rhythm and memory of Three

68

were overwhelming. Carpenter wanted to start building something new at once but knew na was too drunk for that. To sand, imagine, plane, plan, diagram, yes; really build while drunk? Hurt yourself, ruin material, all those things.

Downstairs a Mae West movie was on, fortunately. Carpenter got drunker. Andy was there and carpenter talked to child. Child! Beautiful, solid, real person, Andy. Joy to have been spy on that for fifteen years.

Drunker. Ready to go to bed . . . meaning, nothing to do now but that (two a.m.). In undressing (poured another drink first) for bed carpenter looked in mirror again, swayed again. Carpenter is not unattractive—is attractive—has good strong legs still, belly flat, not too old . . . really unusually attractive body for that age . . . well, listen, no one Three's age is going to turn on by a body of someone your age whatever the condition of the body. True. If I want Three I'll have to play that role——suddenly the carpenter sees that not only is na giving in to counter-revolutionary sex urge but na is also getting ready to play A ROLE TO GET THAT DUCK.

Carpenter is very upset about this and decides to write an article so na can put that kind of behavior on paper (give it to a negative example) and na doesn't naself have to do such a thing.

The carpenter couldn't tell the cook this when na came up the next morning to say, "What did you think of Three?"

So the carpenter was furious at the cook.

The boards lay. The carpenter felt that Saturday morning—alone and unrequired by family, job or movement—erotic. Na thought na would write the article after taking a walk with one of the dogs, doing morning things, getting the day in order. Na could structure the article as na went. Memory of Three surged in halfway down the block; Three pushed in while the dog shat and could not wait for the brief return halfblock to cause that crotch itch. Upstairs,

69

the carpenter took a firm revolutionary view of naself and said out loud: I will turn this eroticism into literature for the movement and not mere self-indulgence via self-orgasm et cetera.

Na knew as na lay on the bed fingers moving toward nan crotch that na loved Three.

8

The afternoon was damp and cold with a grey half-rain that penetrated all the available air by refusing to define itself. The carpenter clung to the garage, the door down and shut from necessity now; na breathed sawdust for air as na sanded board after board, side by side and edge by edge, sanding mechanically in compulsively set and compulsively varied sanding patterns, binding naself.

The cook was alone, left out of love (by all except Stubby whom na could not face, because the cook saw in Stubby's literal body and mind nan own imagination's failure).

The cook lay down on the kitchen floor, as far down as na could get, back straight against the old linoleum. Na stared at the grease and dust coating on the blades of the ceiling fan. Four slanted blades of nan own life, stiff and separate; turning slowly, they would seem to be eight; turning rapidly, they would appear as one almost-transparent disk, through which one unaware would stick a finger to be cut off.

Any moment one of the children could invade. Na closed nan eyes.

I disappear, na willed. Damp hangs in the air and I join it. To mix, knead, cover and set aside dough, let it rise, would bring me inside the dampness. My hands are damp and heavy, the cuptowels are already wet and the floor is sweating. Grey dough bulging in the common way symbolizes humankind—sticky, amorphous, essential. No longer essential: we could live without bread now, we are too well-fed. It is the smell of bread baking that we . . . I crave. To override the chemical stink of a city. Or the convenience of bread for a standing dishless meal, glued slice to slice with peanut butter. The smell is all I could create today. Vapor only. Transient. Single-sensed.

The cook's thoughts pressed into nan mind like the day's air. Na smelled the stale damp of the old linoleum as if its worn-out life were inside nan own head. Na sat up just as the carpenter came in the door.

"What are you doing?"

"I'm reading the labels on our goods," the cook said, standing at the pantry door. "I'm thinking that we can take political theory and package it in different color wrappers with seductive designs, catchy colors, arrange them on shelves in bunches with prices . . . theory may deserve something better but I can't think what today."

The carpenter stood beside na as long as nan own guilt and confusion allowed, nan hand on the cook's shoulder. The cook seemed not to feel it.

"If you can read, you could study each package carefully, learn ingredients and usefulness," the cook said. "But can anyone read in that sense?"

"I'm thinking about writing an article." The carpenter abandoned nan role as shadow and sat down at the table. "I think because I feel abstracted as your labels.

72

The last two days . . . we are very far away from each other, aren't we?"

"I have a feeling our mothers could read the labels, though, and did. But the industry of packaging was newer then. It was probably possible to survey the whole literary field. Weren't half the current ingredients of things on shelves invented and named in the last two decades? Every time a writer writes a label or package-description na invents a new word, right? Nan only creative outlet, after all; why begrudge na. I wonder if it's fair to ask that the invented words be written . . . printed in cerise or aquamarine to distinguish them from the real words? No, what does real mean in such a context?"

"Aren't we?"

"Of course not. I'm just going to bake a cake."

The milk came from a carton decorated with a picture of a cow, the butter was a brick, chocolate in squares, but the eggs for this brand were held in a grey cardboard warren that looked as if raw cardboard had been moistened and molded by a sculptor. The cook held it up to the light, looking into the eggless recesses.

"Raw cardboard? What is that, rags?"

It looked as if it might have been chewed, certainly at least kneaded by delicate fingers before the artist reluctantly shaped it into egg-shaped hollows. There was far more cardboard than necessary, the box was all cardboard hollows except for a thin lid, unlike other egg cartons which let the lid do an inch or two of protection work.

"The sculptor made the cardboard last as long as possible." The cook held it up against the window. Small squares let light through at the corner of each recess, deepening the shadow of the hollow. Even placed finally flat on the counter the cardboard spread its variations like a peacock's tail as na moved about the kitchen.

"It will be an egg cake with variations inspired by the mother container, then," the cook said.

"Godammit, I thought we loved each other," the carpenter shouted. "Can't you even hear me?"

Without a glance at the carpenter, the cook turned on the small radio, settling for the first music station. The carpenter left the kitchen.

The radio sat on the shelf opposite the stove; covered with grease to which dust stuck like tiny flies, it produced its sound unaware. Inside the cook's memory was a thin agile dancing youth left over from fifteen years ago; it now moved torso first into a fantasied dance, feet feeling a centimeter of shift as a yard, arms moving inside, the whole body carrying only its past weight as if the added twenty pounds were laid aside on the counter for the dance.

The cook took out the flour, enormous bin of white so fine it appeared solid, sand of fantasy. It puffed into clouds when transferred bluntly to the sifter, dropped like snow when the sifter turned. The record was changed; Janis Joplin. The dance switched to that beat, arms moving to the plucked guitar and flour falling into hills of powdered sand—drifts of rice-like snow, tiny mountains for powder children. The cake would have that amount of flour needed to complete the landscape to the cook's esthetic satisfaction, the landscape would last as long as that violent pure Texas voice defining freedom reverberated through the mind. The record was over. Salt provided its dent like a brief local rain.

The huge mixer whirled the heavy white batter like lava, creating the same spirals endlessly. Milk, poured in, settled in a spinning crevice constantly closing up around the head of the snake of milk which appeared to be running and pushed back as it grew shorter and shorter and disappeared. Only at the moment it disappeared could the eye see clearly that it was and had been being sucked at from below. But the whirling was monotonous—game to amuse a child. The cook with utter hostility (knowing it was milk) dumped the remainder of the pitcher into the bowl and let the

74

beaters struggle against the assault.

The batter settled into an oblong pan and lay bland and inert. With a skewer the cook placed melted chocolate in small squares around white spaces the size of an egg; the cake would be a negative of the carton. A quick swirl of chocolate discolored each egg space, the hand deciding which should be how dark.

The cook was alone in the kitchen and while the cake baked, danced with huge movements around the center counter spinning the grey and black and dirty cream of the kitchen to fast drums, stamping the ancient floor in faith that no cake could fall when protected by such a massive iron oven, and finally as cake smell began to seep from the oven, lay flat on the floor breathing the too-sweet air, until the music program stopped and na instinctively shut off nan ears before the voice substitute began.

After the cake was done, thin white icing that would harden formed the lid.

"It is better to feel one is the cake," the cook said aloud to no ear. "That it is one's own mind which is being blended by the beaters, given body by the oven, decoration by icing. Then when I ingest my own harmonized mind the circle will be closed."

The carpenter had gone to the living room-dining room-porch space which was undivided and where people from their group and Three and the visitors scattered themselves boundaryless. They played cards, recorders, whittled and talked. Neither Chris nor Leslie were in sight. The carpenter sat near a corner hoping to slump unnoticed.

A sudden brilliant sun broke into the room, clean and alive with color after the day's drizzle. The carpenter let nan eyes look. The room was rich with reflections: trapezoidal streaks across the floor from the windows, spots like stars on the muffin tin and plastic pail, narrow curves outlining the wooden parts of the chairs, thin strips the frames of the doors—on every glass, metal or plastic surface in the room there were irregular integral patches of reflected light. The carpenter looked around the room expressionless. Three was standing near, nan face expectant.

There was no order in light. Light was as near chaos when it reached the earth as the ocean was. This building and its objects interrupted and received light to give it the exact structure it now had. Any object put in light's way would reflect according to its surface and one could not change the pattern of a particular surface reflection—except by moving the object or rearranging the light. Nevertheless it would be silly for the surfaces to feel smug about this, to feel they were important because they reflected in a coherent and characteristic way.

"They just look as if they're behaving intelligently," the carpenter said. "The surfaces, I mean." Na explained.

"That's me too, unfortunately," Three said. "I'm really sorry about last night. I was just high from coming to the sticks and knowing so much, being a movement heavy. It's no excuse; I'm sure old enough to know better. But there it is."

The carpenter's voice was flat. "It's okay. I was a lot older than you before I learned that the rich have feelings too."

"How old do you think I am?" Three asked with the self-conscious half-smile people accompany the question with.

"Twenty-five or so."

"I'm thirty-seven."

The carpenter almost laughed. Looking quickly again at Three, na did laugh. Na stood up and looked again, and laughed again. "I don't believe it!"

"Come on."

"You're thirty-*seven*?"

"What's this age thing with you?"

"It's just that I thought you were a kid." My own

76

kid's age; I didn't want to be the toy of seduction for a kid my own kid's age. "I'm glad though. We're contemporaries, sort of." Relief. I was not completely crazy in thinking about you as a possible . . .

"I don't think age makes any difference."

"Maybe not for people without children. But for us—they're always there to remind us that we're another generation." The carpenter remembered. "But I've always had an age thing. Act your age, I was raised on. I learned to look at all my acts and scenes according to their appropriateness for my age, which meant, I looked at my age daily. I'm responsible for the number of days I've used up this earth's goods; my maturity has to increase proportionately, like pounds on a hog. And forgiveness . . . decreases the same way. For me. For others, it's absolutely obligatory to forgive those with lesser days, which means an unequal relationship. If you were a kid, I'd have to forgive you ubiquitously. We'd have a lopsided friendship. I'd have too much power, you too much freedom which I'd resent when my maturity wasn't well oiled. So I'm glad you're near my age. I'm forty-three."

"Of course our backgrounds are pretty lopsided. And our hair isn't the same color."

"I wasn't looking for a twin."

"I know. I'm glad you're looking for a friend." Three grinned. "So I get six years worth of forgiveness. Suppose I need more than that? But the power thing is interesting: most people in the movement are coupled up with people their own height, more than anything. Size and weight about the same. It's a question of who's going to win in the showdown fight, who can beat up who. That's where the power has always been."

"Thanks for skipping over the pocketbook."

"It was a high skip. But you're tall too."

"I get it either way," the carpenter said distractedly. Na was preoccupied by the cook's refusal to talk, by nan anger which the carpenter did not understand. Na moved toward the kitchen. Three saw the imprint of

77

trouble on the carpenter's face; as the carpenter excused naself to go back to the kitchen, na saw that Three saw.

"A friendship like yours," Three nodded toward the kitchen, "can survive a fight. That's for sure."

"No. You see, I love na." The hardest statement for the carpenter to make ever was easier, now that it was not exactly true. Inside the kitchen, the cake was not in sight.

"Did you eat it?" the carpenter asked that night— a half-stupid question: creators are not usually consumers. But if the fancy commercial bakers . . . "You ate it!" The carpenter kissed the top of the cook's head. "Because that's what you would do— it's the courage to extricate oneself from the cliche. Right? If the fancy commercial bakers, as proud of their roses as an English gardener, regard their creations as a product then you, involved only in the act of making a cake, might easily simply eat it. The really creative act."

"It was the most beautiful experience of my life because I *made* that cake. Look"—a long oblique look at the sky beyond the ceiling—"I've never made a cake before. To really cook you have to feel each thing you put in. If we cooked that way, everybody, cooking would have the complexities and soul of art . . . but better because art is useless as a product. But the human stomach and the cook-artist—now there's the perfect combination for a real consumer and an artist with a product." The cook frowned. "Of course all that does is give you a goal in present psychological terminology. But the art part . . . you see, you take meaningless unrelated raw materials and up them together according to the moment's music and the unexpressed dance hidden inside your own body . . ."

"You ate it!" the carpenter said with a skip.

"No. You aren't understanding me. What I mean

78

is that sometimes forging into new territory or allowing yourself new boundaries preserves your sanity but then you have to live in them and that's entirely different. Maybe too hard. I was afraid that where I had been—making that cake—was a pinnacle of the mind on which I could balance for a minute but not live. I had to come back down."

After the cook left the carpenter released the impatient anger caused by the cook's last retreat. "I do understand. But at your rate it will take much too long to reach your own ultimate limits—or nonlimits. Much too long." The carpenter paced the floor and mentally raced ahead in imagination searching for a possible structure which could express the anger and also release the cook from that fear. A triangulated hinged Moebius strip to exterpolate insanity into its final form? No, a structure of interlocked boxes, a beehive in octagons, offered to the cook as a container for unusual spices . . . a totally intricate web of shapes which . . . no. It should be built big enough for children to play in, a cubistic Moebius strip which the child could crawl around over any surface and never get anywhere, like a Hansel and Gretel dropping crumbs over their past becoming future. An intellectual squirrel cage . . .

The carpenter worked on it for a week and called the cook to come and see.
"It's subtle, beautiful! It's like a new word." The cook's face glowed during a long minute examination of each angle and plane. "Really beautiful. A new word." The carpenter felt suddenly united with nan love in an invasion of pleasure.
Later though, during a pause in the conversation which coincided with an eerie soundlessness in the house itself, the carpenter saw something else struggling under the surface of the cook's face. An objection.

"You don't like something about it, though."

"I was wondering, yes," the cook said softly. "That this may be the male copout, the structure that teases emotion, equivocates the impulse to grow . . . to open completely to each other. A structure which a child would know enough to refuse to enjoy because to find joy in such a complicated abstraction would be to betray simplicity, the god of childhood."

"You think I made it to tease you?"

The cook answered obliquely. "Your hostility comes out in unique ways. We are committed to honesty and I would have to mistrust an absence of anger, but this is superstructured anger masquerading as creativity. But maybe that's what creativity is." The lilt in the last sentence was just off center, catching on some denial underneath, missing smoothness.

The carpenter focussed on the cook's face, trying to isolate the denial. "It is possible that I might think that sometimes but impossible that you could. Either you are becoming me or you're being soothing, for christsakes."

"Right." The cook's eyes were dark and intense. "I wouldn't want to sidestep anything."

"Sidestep what? Fuck it. You divide up like mercury when I want to talk about why we're not close and what happened. You slip off into your own creativity and bake a cake and when I try to do the same thing you call it a goddamn costume party."

"I had to. Maybe you had to too and weren't just following me. But you know why we're not close. What happened."

"What?" The carpenter's face was flushed with anger and knowledge.

"When I was able to make that cake I was telling you that you have given me the courage to act with the freedom I've always wanted. You answer, 'Love is sleeping together,' and say you want to nibble my right ear. It's the left, I say—but neither of us is talking about love."

80

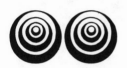

9

One night the carpenter and Three lay in each other's arms and loved each other entirely until morning.

The next day all day the strong unique smell of Three remained, blowing suddenly through the field where the carpenter walked as if the entire earth were inside nan nose's memory.

I close my eyes and see your eyes, deep brown flecked with yellow, brown-yellow flecks like strange under-parts of the sea where fish are seen only by you looking for fish, cropping bubbles at each unheard pause. We curved in and out of each other as if our bodies themselves were sea-water. How extraordinary to have held you for an entire night!

The carpenter lay on the grass, the tender side of nan body remembering. Your body crumpled into mine as if each of our bumps and hollows were negatives of the other's, as if we were made of silly putty taking the

83

shape of our container at each pressure point . . . as if, darling, we were lovers. I held your body effortlessly but I thought that I alone supported it from falling forever down or outward. You filled my vacant places with the tenderness I have felt only when holding my own baby infant. Yet you are not my child, you are the tenderness. You are not a child at all but you bring to us the vibrancy of child, the ability to make the two of us complete within an irrelevant world.

There was a sensuous, warm, slightly hungry heat of awareness inside nan back muscles, in nan stomach and mouth, joining into a focus at nan throat. The carpenter was suspended in the mysteriousness of being alive, total heightened experience as if na were a visitor to the past (today). Privilege of temporary return to this day from the distant future; from death. Na saw the now as one would see a lost culture if abruptly deposited there . . . mystery of every detail; nan own presence unremarked. How did I get here? where was I before? how long will I be able to stay? But these thoughts themselves seemed to have been translated into the language of this past country: in nan mind there was no expression for "how long," as if time had no length-component at all. Each square-root of a second vibrated and was utterly without the old characteristic of seconds—the sense within themselves that another second would follow. These seconds existed as drops of life suspended in space. Na visited them separately.

"I don't have a self," the carpenter said aloud. The word *self* echoed through nan mind as if the mind were a conch shell. The sound of *self* had the shape and rubbed smoothness of the conch . . . say it over, hear as a child hears . . . elf introduced with a whisper.

November. Three and the carpenter had just returned from a meeting at the Mexican-American center. They had met, not the people as they had planned, but their "leader." The carpenter had been allowed to read a paper, translated into Spanish by Stubby, explaining what their group was doing and inviting any of the people present to join them, use them, whatever. After a brief question period (translated by the "leader"), Three and the carpenter had been shuffled into a side room where the same self-appointed leader had explained everything to them—explained what two thousand people wanted or needed. They had made no contact with the people at all.

All the way home on the bus they had talked, alternately angry and depressed. Three's anger was raging by the time they reached the house.

"That son of a chicken snake wants to run for city council—that's all na is about," Three said. "And that's the last any poor person is going to see of na until na pops up on the other side of friendly finance with the poor slob's car in nan mouth. If na thinks na is going to get my support just because na speaks Spanish and has a batch of desperate Mexicans hanging off nan shirtfront . . . can't they see what na is about? There's no dialogue, no interchange, no two-way—na tells them what na is going to do for them and that's about as much as the manufacturers of Carta Blanca." They sat on the glider on the deck the carpenter had sanded and stained, the gentle slip of the glider beginning to temper Three's anger. "We lost it because we can't speak Spanish. That's the power that leader has."

The carpenter was silent. Na could speak Spanish but did not dare. Na felt na was too blond to use the language openly. If na had been Three, na would have spoken; the contact they had wanted would have been made.

"That pig bragging about adopting an orphan. Thirteen! 'So beautiful,' " Three mimicked. "It's fucking obvious what that charity is about. *Pig*."

"Look," the carpenter said. "I can speak Spanish, a little."

"You can?"

"I was too scared to. I know I should have but I just couldn't."

Three touched the carpenter's hair, cupping nan head as if it were an exhibit. "Why not?" Anger had disappeared from nan voice. "You've got more brains than any leader, than anyone I know. You could have . . . listen, did you understand what the people were saying?"

"The leader twisted the questions," the carpenter said.

"I knew it!"

"Na made it as if they were asking something just off what they meant. I'm really angry at myself . . ."

"It was that room. That stage, all those rows of chairs. Could you talk if there was just one or two people? We can go again!" The possibility banished anger altogether. "You can speak Spanish! Is there anything you can't do, my perfect harp?"

The carpenter watched a fingernail moon dart in and out of clouds. "Tell me something. Did you really mean what you said last night, that I escape definition?" Three nodded. It was the carpenter's fantasy about naself, the one thing na most wanted to be—a non-be, in a sense; completely fluid. The carpenter's hands, large and knobby, described now in the air for Three nan own most deeply felt belief in chaos. The reason na had become a carpenter was the lust of nan hands to touch, grasp, caress, move or change the shape of whatever was accessible. To see what structures could be dissolved but also to restructure in wood and nails—geometrically, to organize space, interrupt air, because in this way the mind could remain chaotic and could even be balanced, ballasted, protected by putting the structures into the room not in the mind. Because a mind not in a state of chaos was a pecan dented and pressed by a shell, shell resting in every groove. "Take water from the ocean and hold it in a jar," the carpenter said. "It is chemically-defined ocean only; all the essential ocean attributes of movement and white noise and meaning are lost. I remember when my mind was structured, imprisoned in the time my body happened

86

to be born, its thoughts impaled on the language of that structure-system. I was still wriggling too when the cook and I were together—we were people with histories, of a certain age. You know. Caught behind a jut of earth. Still seeing things in pros or cons, this or that, *a* versus *b*—opposites. But with you . . ." The carpenter's hands stopped, lit on Three's knee, held nan arm to force touch to transmit understanding. "It's not at all that you are a third possibility, it's that you are all three at once—plus, minus and other. You are three if three is a perfect circle of all possibilities. Do you understand what I mean?"

Three freed nan arm and encircled the carpenter's head, bending nan face to nan own. "I know that together we have gone beyond anything I've ever known," na said, kissing the carpenter's cheek with the words.

10

By January the group felt itself together enough to act. Some of them were angry that they had had to wait this long. The Christmas holidays, in particular, had left the atmosphere around the house permeated with past emotions, with the world they had discarded but which the children and their own memories could not quite. The most impatient felt that the air should be cleared at once.

Regular cleaning day was Sunday.

"It's New Year's Eve," Three said.

"Perfect," the carpenter said.

"Aren't we going to have a New Year's Eve party?" Andy said. Andy was still fifteen.

"You can have a beer while you sweep," Tracy said. Tracy had attached naself like a barnacle onto the carpenter and Three, nan writer's instinct gluing itself to the center of whatever was to happen.

"It's wonderful how much time we spend pleasing our eyes," the cook said. "I wonder if the blind bother to do housework?" The cook poked a finger at Andy. "You chillen can have a party if you want to since you're not old enough to know what an anti-party is. Neither am I. I'll even go get your hooch for you."

"Can we have champagne?" Andy said.

"In the middle of the revolution?"

"Next thing, they'll want cake."

"I'm not baking," the cook said. "When I clean I don't mess, when I mess . . ."

"Oh, we don't need food," Andy said and ran off to tell the others.

"Take Nicky with you," the cook called after na. "I'm happy because Nicky, total materialist, has spent the whole week counting presents. Na is so afraid na'll forget what number na is at that na doesn't dare break concentration to shout all those obscenities. It's telling on na, though. I heard na counting yesterday: one-shit, two-shit, three-shit."

"I won't take it personally," Three said.

"I'm chewing Andy's gum!" Tracy held out a wad of grey na had taken from nan mouth. "It's the first time I've had someone else's gum in my mouth since I was a kid. My brother used to do that, play 'swap gum,' until Mother found out and made us stop it. It's that slightly-foreign saliva slipping over your mouth from someone else's mouth . . . Andy put nan gum into the ashtray where I usually put mine—I told na to put it there. I often pick up my gum later. You get tired of chewing it, put it down, pick it up later to chew some more. It's not the flavor your mouth wants but a container for your own saliva. Andy's gum was juicy fruit—it was the first taste of juicy fruit that told me it was Andy's gum. My gum is always mint. But I can't believe I'm chewing Andy's gum."

"We're all into each other's spit," the cook said. "But as long as Mother plays policeman everything's going to be all right; just the same."

89

"Did you know *spit* means *image*?" the carpenter said. "In *spit and image*: it's just another word for image."

"Throw some soapsuds at me," Three said. "I'm dry over here."

"You're on the Baptist part of the floor," the cook said. "You believe."

"All phosphate but I believe it's soap," Three said.

"Nobody knows the houses I've cleaned," the cook sang. "If the generals had to wash up all the blood they spilled, do you think we'd have war?"

"If the presidents had to pick up their own socks and wash them, make up their beds, think about their own meals, they wouldn't become so abstract," the carpenter said.

"How come you're so abstract?" Three said.

"That's how I know. I'm learning though." The carpenter picked up a boxful of plastic play-pieces. "All the games those people play when they're children deal with their boredom. They grow up and are still bored because they don't have anything useful to do, so they play the same games—Tonka toys, tin soldiers, monopoly. They don't even have to put the earth or the nations or the cities back when they're through. You know who picks up after them."

The cook said, "You make a joke around here and someone turns it into a theory. I was just kidding about the generals."

"You were?" The carpenter held the mop in front and moved closer to the cook, mop threatening nan stomach. "But you said a very important thing. You know what the squatters said about New York? 'The rich play monopoly with New York City while the poor go directly to jail.'"

"Did they say that?" Three said. "That's good."

"No, I made it up. But it's true," the carpenter said. "It's always a game when you don't have to provide your own toilet paper. Did I ever tell you about the dream I had about the washing machine? I dreamed

90

that the washing machine was broken, all the pieces were separating from each other, so I held it together while the clothes washed. It took twice as much time and strength to hold the machine together like that as it would have just to wash the clothes by hand. But I held it together load after load. Why did I do that?"

Three burst out laughing. "We're going to elect you president. That's what they do."

"We sure eat a lot," the cook said. "We eat everywhere. By this couch, there's peanut butter, used dixie cups, a chocolate milk carton, a wrapper from a package of orioles and a box of sugar pops dregs." Another swipe of the broom brought out a roll of glass . . . "And here're the peanuts. Do you think the president's house looks like this?"

By eight-fifteen Monday the meeting was ready to begin.

"I think we should choose someone to chair this meeting," the carpenter said. "The last one was chaos. Now I like chaos myself but we have a lot to talk about. Anyone object? Okay. Ten."

"Twenty-five," Tracy said.

"Whose birthday is in October nearest the twenty-fifth?"

"That's my birthday!" Nicky said.

"You're the chair then."

"Okay." Nicky grinned and scooted still cross-legged across the floor until na was in the center of the circle. "What's the meeting about?"

"It's about . . ."

"Hold up your fucking hand and wait till you're recognized," Nicky said. "Okay, carp."

"We have to try to clarify the nature of the thing we want to establish—is it going to be more of a center or more of a school, and what do we want to call it. Then, should we take over a building or settle for using the house we have. And what projects do people have already planned for the center or school or want to start. I guess we have to talk about them all at once since they depend on each other."

"Good," Nicky said. "Next?"

"Skip the applause," the cook said.

"Three?"

"I've been going to city council meetings and school board meetings and budget hearings besides a lot of honky tonks and I know three buildings this town is sitting on that they took away from the people and I think we ought to help them out of one-third of that mistake at least. I think we ought to call it a center because what I'd like to see is a place where we can get together to rap and support each other. We can have a hot-line for people who freak out because the principal threw them out of school or the cops busted them or the boss fired them. And I'd like to set up an alternate to that pig-run bar over on Fig Tree Street. That's the name of the street. Whatever we call this center, I know what it is: it's a revolution against the slave-family, the slave-house, the slave-bed and the whole copulating system."

"Leslie?"

"I think we should think about it first before we come out strong against marriage and the family. The black people in town . . . marriage is a kind of status thing with us because we've always been put down for not getting married and not having stable families and all."

"Yeah, that's true," the cook said. "If we want the freedom to work out our own way of doing things, we have to allow others the freedom to choose family or marriage. I think . . ."

"You want to be recognized?" Nicky said. "Okay, you are."

"I think I prefer to call it—whatever it is—a school rather than a center but that's mainly because I like words of one syllable when possible."

"Down here 'school' has two syllables too," Andy said. "Schoo-uhl."

"Right."

92

"I want to say something," Stubby said. "We've just conceded our first compromise: we allow the blacks to eliminate our taking a stand on marriage because it would alienate some of the people we're trying to reach. Then by what logic will you not allow us to eliminate the stand on homosexuality because it will alienate some people we're trying to reach? And it sure as hell will."

"Can I answer that?" Tracy said. "Okay. Freedom of sexual choice is absolutely basic; marriage is just one issue. Freedom of sexual choice includes marriage— and third-world people. If people have to tie themselves up in wedding knots because that's where their heads are at, we're not going to try to stop them. We're going to be there to help when they start strangling."

"But it's still true that every time a black person asks for a compromise, we say sure. Every time a middle-class white asks the same thing, we put na down for being uptight. It's like we valued black members more than white ones." The cook stopped before the chair got na.

"Right," Stubby said.

"We're afraid of that criticism: you're nothing but a white middle-class movement," the carpenter said. "That's what gets to us. That really hurts more than the other criticism: you're nothing but a bunch of queers."

"The reason that other criticism doesn't hurt any more is because the queers stood up to it," Three said. "Everybody said, sure we are and we're beautiful. You tell 'em and you shut 'em up."

"Now I ask you," Stubby said. "How can a middle-class white stand up and say, sure I am and I'm beautiful? After what the media has done to that term?"

"Maybe that's the point. Maybe we should say just that," the cook said.

"But everyone probably has some homosexuality in them and that's one reason the other tactic worked.

93

Everyone doesn't have some middle-class white in them: the blacks for instance," Stubby said.

"Yes, they do," Leslie said.

"There's a difference," the carpenter said. "The third-world people see the white middle class as an enemy trying to destroy their jobs, homes, schools and identities. No one has ever complimented the homosexual movement by giving it that kind of status. No one has seen homosexuals as much of a threat at all, except as individuals challenging individuals. Maybe it's a real threat or can become one, but right now it's not an organized power group. That's the difference. One doesn't even have to know homosexuality exists. You can't say that about the white middle class."

"I'm against any compromise on the homosexual issue because that's the very basis of freedom," Tracy said. "I know I said that before. But as long as large groups of people are considered only as sexual commodities and their whole livelihood depends on them being that . . . they can't make a decent living in this society without using that. That's what marriage is, that people can trade their value as sexual commodities for support. It's probably less true though in most third-world marriages than in middle-class white ones, because in the former both partners work. But as long as everyone sees as a higher value that only one partner should work for money and the other should work (usually much harder) for so-called love . . . then the working classes are just as deluded as anyone. They're headed in the same direction—upward which is really downward. I don't think we should agree to compromise on the marriage issue, either."

"We'll have everyone against us," Stubby said.

"That's better than getting people to join us under false pretenses," Tracy said.

"People need time to change their ways of thinking on such basic issues. My god," Stubby said.

"Who's rushing them? They can take all the time

they want to stand back and listen to us or watch us. They don't have to join us until they're ready. They shouldn't," Tracy said.

"Shut up," Nicky said. "You two are talking too much."

"Let's go around the room," the carpenter said. "Chris?"

"I wish we didn't always get back to class and money," Chris said, "I don't think we should compromise on the homosexual issue at all because there are homosexuals in this town who need our support. That's the main thing. We have to reach out to them. And to everybody who needs our support—people who're for marriage, people who are against it, all kinds. I just think we should think in terms of people—individuals wherever they are—not in generalities about society and stuff where I can't tell one person's argument from the other's."

"Just so we don't shut out married people," Leslie said. "I guess I'm thinking about my parents. But they got to learn too. Anyway, they're not here."

Meredith from the theater group was recognized and stood up. "Okay. I just want to say one thing: I think we've all lost our minds. Here—in this place where the white-black issue . . . intermarriage, mixing up the races, is the biggest threat these people know, we're going to eliminate the male-female? Expect them to accept homosexuality? It's insane."

"Why?" Three said. "Keep the races pure that way."

"You're out of your mind," Meredith said.

"Let's get on to the projects," the carpenter said.

"Who wants the floor?" Nicky said. "Ask, don't grab."

"We do," Carter said. "The health project is ready to go and we don't care whether we work under the title of center or school, we don't care whether the people who come to us are married or homosexual or both—but we're not going to pretend to believe anything we don't believe. Whatever that is. We've gotten a lot of

95

promises from the community around here for support, and some firm commitments. We need one doctor to be legal and we have two who have promised to be on call—one or the other of them—at all times and to give us certain hours every week. We have the equipment for simple tests and plenty of free literature to start classes with. The thing is we figure we need at least three rooms and at least one of them should have a street entrance. The waiting room, probably. We don't want people to have to wander all over a strange building to find us when they are sick or upset. Then we need a private room for treatment off that and a room where the children can be entertained if parents have to bring them. We really need more and different space than this house has so we're for getting another building any way we can get it. There are three of us—besides me, there's Bert and Norton. If anyone . . ."

"Me," Leslie said.

"There's Leslie," Chris said.

"And Leslie. And anyone else who wants to help or join is welcome. And we're ready to go right now."

"Right on."

"Beautiful."

"Can the applause," Nicky said. "Next?"

Chris said, "Well, this isn't really together yet, but some of us want to start getting into our own bodies, with dance and movement if the cook'll help, and street-fighting and things like that too. There are a couple of kids at school who're interested. We'll set up regular times to meet and see what happens, see what we can learn from each other, but the way we see it, pretty soon it'll be happening all the time wherever we are, not just in the hours we meet. I hope that's clear but I don't think it is." Chris stopped. "Oh yes, I forgot. We all want to work on building maintenance too. I want to learn plumbing and there's a kid at school who said na would teach us."

"Next?"

Meredith stood up. "The theater group is myself and Jesse and Bren. We also double or overlap with the art group—that's the cook. We'd like to make leaflets and posters and things like that. We don't care where we are . . . could you please save the private conversations until after the meeting? I mean, we'd like a whole building of course but we'll play off the sidewalk if we have to. We want to have theater actions all over town, especially weekends and especially for children and teenagers. We've been working on publicity and we think we can get good press coverage. One of us is dating a local reporter to make sure we do, in fact. We can . . . maybe no one is interested in this," na said angrily and waited. The whispering stopped.

"Yes, we are."

"Go on."

"Shhhh."

"Shhhh."

"I simply refuse to try to outshout people who don't have the courtesy to keep quiet even if they don't want to listen." Meredith's face quivered as if na were being booed and jeered by a theater audience. There was silence in the room. "I won't take up any more time than I have to. A fifth grade teacher from the Fairgrounds elementary school wants to join us, and two teachers from the Chocolate Creek elementary school —first and third grade. They're really interested and will bring their classes to the first play. What? Yes, that's the black school. They're trying to change the name. We've had less success in the junior high schools. We have one promise from the art teacher at Robert E. Lee but na is new this year and still cautious. I doubt if na will get involved until na sees how the town takes it. None of us can speak Spanish but Stubby said na would work with us and teach us the words we know we'll be saying and be there to translate when we ad lib, as we usually do. We try to keep the plays mostly action anyway. That's about all. There is more but people obviously aren't in the mood to hear it. What?"

"What about us?" Nicky said.

"Oh, yes. Besides the people I named, most of the children are also a part of this group. Thank you for reminding me, Nicky. Nicky is one, and Andy and Kirby and . . ."

"I'm not," Andy said.

"But you were this morning," Meredith said.

"I'm not now. I want to be with Chris and the street-fighting."

"Well, of course." Meredith stopped, nan face flushed and trembling.

"Sweeper?" Nicky said.

Sweeper leaned forward and grinned. Na was from the town, had lived there all na life. Na was recently divorced and had joined the group a month before with nan two children. "We've got the greatest child-care set-up that ever came down the pike. We've . . ."

"Wait a minute, please. I'm sorry, but wait just a minute," Meredith said. "I have to say something first. There is a definite feeling of hostility in this room tonight and I want to know what it's about. Apparently it has to do with me. First there's the whispering, then there's the continued whispering after I asked you to stop . . . do you have any idea how rude it is to whisper while someone is trying to talk? Then there's Andy suddenly dissociating naself from a group na was a member of this morning as far as I know. Now I want to know what this is about. If anyone has anything to say against me, say it now."

"I just don't want to any more," Andy said, near tears.

"Na has a right to . . ." Chris began angrily.

"May I have the floor?" Stubby stood up and took it. "I must say I know what Meredith is talking about. It's not you, Andy. There is now and has been from the beginning certain factions—yes, that's the word—in this group who deliberately foster dissent and antagonism . . ."

"Hold it," Carter said. "Stop right there. Now back

98

up behind 'deliberately' and start over or I'm not going to let you say another word."

"It's only fair that I be allowed to use the words I choose," Stubby said.

"What's this appeal to bourgeois democracy?" Three said.

"I think I can tell Meredith where the hostility is coming from," the cook said. "The children were an after-thought. They thought they were a part of the group and they didn't expect to be treated like that here. We all know they're treated like that everywhere else. But when you named the members of the theater group you just named the adults and Nicky had to remind you about the kids. That's the main thing. But the other thing is the way you talked about the press—like we were still into dating games to get our pictures in the paper. Maybe we're still not sure that we're not and that's why it's offensive."

"Thank you for telling me," Meredith said. "I mean that. I appreciate it that someone has the guts to speak right out and tell me, instead of whispering behind my back. I'm sorry about the children. You're absolutely right, it was inexcusable. I apologize and it won't happen again. Of course they are just as much a part of the group as anyone else. I don't understand what you mean about the press, though. I thought we wanted media coverage. We were led to believe . . ."

"We absolutely and unequivocally do," Stubby said. "Believe me, there is no point in doing any action at all if the press isn't there. It won't be communicated to anyone. It's essential to have the press and I don't care how we get them."

"I do."

"I'm sure not going to peddle my ass for any story."

"Fuck the press. They'll put us on the children's page anyway."

"I think we should save the media for another meeting. It's already late."

"Go on, Sweeper," Nicky said.

"We've got the greatest childcare plan that ever came down the pike . . ."

Leslie's eyes were closed and nan face upturned to the moon. "Something's wrong. It hit me when I said, 'my parents.' I started thinking about them."

"I figured that was it," Chris said.

Leslie looked at Chris. The moonlight was now on nan hair, glistening like a shield over nan face. "I've got to stand for something. Right now I feel like a tangle of bits of string. Now am I supposed to identify with the oppressed gay people or the oppressed black people, with the middle class my people are in or the working class my other people are in, with the kids I just barely left or the parents I'm supposed to become, with the city I grew up in or the community I choose to live in . . . I could go on forever." The night was cold and Leslie shivered. "I could divide myself up by race or class or sex or money or age or past or future. Shit man, I'm a fucking rat's nest of oppressed parts."

Sweeper wore the dress of the town, light colors and cotton shirts which never acknowledged the existence of the short winter. There was democracy in the way the people all dressed the same, and stability in the lack of seasons.

Sweeper did not understand the political arguments. "We all want the same thing, what's the use of fighting each other?" na said to Stubby when the meeting broke up. "You're just like me and I know I'm mainly scared of people not liking me. That's why I say asinine things sometimes. Sometimes I'll say just about anything to get people to like me, to be one of everybody." Na laughed. "Then I swear up and down that I won't be so miserably wishy-washy next time, and then next time I do it again. It's because deep down you really like people too much, you care too much."

Stubby's face showed the under-prod of the sentence

na longed to blurt out: I don't like people at all; couldn't care less. Na compromised with, "We shouldn't get overinvolved in our own private needs and forget that we have work to do."

Sweeper said quickly, "I'm not fussing at you." Nan eyes were wide with Texas plenty. "I'm much worse. I'm the one who's silly about it. You're naturally more serious and that's why it hurts you so much when people . . . I mean you say what you believe, never mind whether anybody likes it, much more than I ever could, and it hurts when they don't respect you for it. You think they don't. They really do."

Stubby's anger was about to erupt. "I don't respect them for deliberately trying to turn this whole town against us."

"Now you don't mean that!"

"I just don't understand Stubby," Sweeper said later to Tracy.

Tracy had been searching for the words with which to make a portrait of Stubby ever since the meeting. Na had come up with a tentative one and tried it out on Sweeper. "It's not that what Stubby says is so wrong, not that. It's nan face that looks like it is making a speech. There is an absence of reaching out in nan expression, a clippedness to nan hair which makes na look as if somehow nan eyes and mouth were also carefully trimmed."

Sweeper looked puzzled. "I think I see what you mean. But when you're stout, you know, you try harder to be neat. I know I ought to."

"That's not what I meant," Tracy said.

Sweeper's round eyes were apologetic. "I don't get it but I know you're right. You're all too smart for me."

Andy was sharing a cigarette with Nicky on the back stoop. "You're the best chair we ever had," Andy said.

"I tried to shut them up," Nicky said. "Some people always talk. It makes me feel stupid."

101

"Balls," Andy said. "They don't know what they're trying to say either. They act like they think they might remember if they talk long enough."

The carpenter walked beside Three without listening. Na was occupied with the sense and image of the cook and the cold wind that blew from the cook's words to the carpenter's earlier love for na, now crowding back into the carpenter's chest like sandcrabs into a beach. The carpenter felt that the cook was speaking directly into nan soul. I am hiding by the side of the revolution hoping to be ridden and included. I should shout instead: I am a middle-class white, try and stop me. One can doubt the wisdom of any issue, but to lose contact with the person whom one was once closest to, is to be free and clear of any doubt—is to be clearly wrong and free for nothing.

Na said to Three, "We have to take over a building. Before we talk ourselves apart."

Meredith's nostrils were flared with the fury of a wild horse. Carter hardly knew Meredith but now na responded to the visible pounding of nan anger.

"When people criticize you in a meeting, it's hard not to take it personally," Carter said. "I know for me the worst moment I had in the movement was when I suddenly felt that right here, in the middle of a meeting, I had nothing but enemies. Then what did I have anywhere else?"

"I don't understand why everyone is against Stubby," Meredith said, projecting nan voice as if from a stage. "My god, na does half the work that ever gets done around here. Stubby is one of the few who really seems to care about getting this group off its ass and into doing something. What the hell is the matter with that?"

"For one thing, na wants us to do what na tells us to do. Na interrupts when the group is trying to work out together what it wants to do. For another, one person doing other people's share of the work is always demoralizing and sometimes a way of making oneself indispensable in order to gain power."

"Save us," Meredith said, nan eyes flashing. "You don't think . . ."

"It crosses my mind," Carter said quietly. "On its way to other minds, I feel sure."

"That's insane," Meredith said, but nan face grew thoughtful.

The cook felt the sense of loss, sense without a name that has to be described by metaphor, sense of the sun shining one hour after an unremittingly grey week and then disappearing . . . sun reminding us of what we have missed, teasing us by vacating the window an hour before dark, leaving our last day-hour greyer by far than any of the week prior. Loss like that of a bird's death—bird you had saved, injured bird which had cried into your life, broken all your patterns with its helplessness . . . you held it like your own lost beginnings, held your breath at the delicacy of its life, placed it carefully in the box you built and gave it water and worms and sought books in the library to understand its kind; for two days all your energy and thought went into persuading it to live. It died. Then it is the kind of loss that includes the feeling that one has been tricked; we were better off before, not seeing the sun at all, not opening up to the fragility of the bird. The cook felt this.

Partly because when Nicky became chair of the meeting that burden lifted and the cook felt suddenly lighter—too much lighter, na would lift off the floor. To be so light was to be companionless.

But primarily because the cook felt silence through all the words.

103

11

The carpenter was at work at seven one morning. Na heard nothing there inside nan own concentration and jumped when na saw the pair of feet beside the pine plank.

"I didn't mean to scare you." The cook's skin glowed from the crisp clear morning air but nan eyes slipped sideways each time the carpenter's met them. The cook had brought coffee for both of them. The carpenter put a clean piece of board over the sawdust. They sat side by side. The carpenter blew across the hot coffee and steam covered nan glasses.

"Thanks for the coffee," the carpenter said. "That's really nice of you."

"I had to get away from the kids," the cook said. Na hoped the carpenter understood. It was a line from a poem. It meant, kids are just kids, after all. It meant, I've been wrong all the time, using the kids as a closet.

Busy work. Make you feel important. I've been disappearing into the kids. Safe there. Na looked at the carpenter's face to see if na understood. "See?"

"Sure," the carpenter said, waiting.

The cook needed more time. "It's a beautiful morning!" na said in the voice of a bird. "Isn't it?" And then, after a moment, "What are you making?"

"I'm really glad you came," the carpenter said.

"Oh." The cook fumbled for a cigarette. "What *are* you making?"

The carpenter explained. The garage na was remodelling . . . they wanted a heavy desk, two doors actually, laid end to end, extremely heavy doors. They wanted it hung from the wall with no legs. The carpenter had worked out a support, five triangles, isosceles so the thrust of the weight would be directed back against the garage uprights. The top two by fours were used flat, the hypotenuse two by fours skinnyways, and a cut made in the flat of the top support to receive the hypotenuse's tip (sliced horizontal, of course). "Then I drilled a hole through both boards and put a bolt through to hold that angle. That was the hardest part—to drill from both sides since my bit isn't long enough to go all the way through. Drills should be made with a leveller on them so you could be sure you were always perpendicular." The cook's presence was so immediate in the open vacuum of pre-morning that the carpenter's ears set up their ringing at "perpendicular." The cook's eyes would meet nan's only for a second.

The cook bent earnestly over the angle described. Morning sun caught the flying strands of hair like dew. "How long is the bit?" na said. Na picked it up and held it across a two by four. It was a quarter-inch short. Less. Nan own bit-sized fingers measured the flattened shaft that was inserted in the drill. "Couldn't you not stick the shaft all the way in?"

The ringing abruptly stopped as the carpenter suddenly saw. "You're a genius!" Na hugged the cook. "You solved the problem. You are a genius."

105

The cook was brushing coffee off nan sweater. "Then it's worth losing all that coffee."

"I'm sorry. Have some of mine." The carpenter poured half nan coffee into the cook's cup, sloshing it over the cook's hand and shoes.

"Forget that." The cook held the carpenter's hand to prevent na from bending down to wipe off the shoes. "The coffee was only for show." The carpenter shivered as their eyes met; na forced the ringing away. "I wanted to tell you something," the cook said. "The summer after the baby was born, we spent a week at an apartment in Queens. It belonged to my sister's husband's mother—na had to go into the hospital in New York and nan husband suggested we trade apartments so na could be near na. They lived in a huge apartment complex with a lot of grass. In the middle of August I thought it was paradise. The first night we were there I went outside to walk barefoot in that grass. Then I was running and leaping—it was so soft and alive—and I cut my foot wide open on a broken bottle. I felt more betrayed than anything. How could that green velvet be hiding a broken beer bottle? I had to walk sideways on the foot the next day. But it got infected anyway. Doctor told me to stay off it. 'Keep it up,' he said. Keep it up and I'll kill myself next, I thought. 'Keep what up, my chin?' I said. He meant that too. Well, I thought, the children have the grass, they should be able to manage their meals in return for that. They only ate peanut butter and cereal anyway. They managed—they even managed to get some food down the baby. They let na climb up to the table and pour milk in nan own cereal so it was all over the table, the bench, and was padded across the linoleum and out the door. Well, so the time came when I asked one of them to bring me a glass of milk. 'Aw gee, I did it last time. Ask Nicky,' na said. 'Bullshit. I did it last time,' Nicky yelled. They both disappeared. I asked Terry. 'It's not my turn,' na whined. That's what I get, I thought. Imagine a parent asking a child for a glass of

106

milk. Milk only goes in the other direction. I knew it all the time but I couldn't believe it. I started keeping a diary, writing it all down. I didn't want to forget again. 'Not me!' 'You always ask me, never Nicky!' 'It's Terry's turn!' 'Your old foot's all right. You're just using that as an excuse to make us wait on you.' Then I'd hear them in the next room, imitating me. 'You're trying to drive me crazy,' one of them would mimic. 'Crazy. After all I've done for you.'

"All week I kept my foot up and got it all down. I swore I'd never forget it. But I did." The cook hesitated, then asked softly, "Do you understand what I'm trying to tell you?"

The carpenter understood. Na nodded. Na reached for the cook's hand, changed the impulse to hold into a pat, pulled nan hand back. Na felt split down the middle. It's timing, naself told naself. Think. Think. "I . . . I mean, it's not . . . you see . . . Look. I think I know what you're saying. But . . ."

The cook stood up. "I just wanted you to know. I'm not asking you to do anything. Just know." Na picked up the coffee cups. "I hope the drill thing works."

The carpenter moved quickly to open the door, to block nan exit a moment. "Thanks. For the solution, too, but thanks mainly for coming."

Timing.

The night before Three had returned from a trip to the city. Na had been gone a week, but it was not just the absence that made the carpenter especially want to see na; Three and the carpenter had had several arguments prior to the trip and their relationship was shaky.

The final argument, the night before Three left, remained in the carpenter's head all week. The carpenter could not go on the trip with Three because na had work to finish; nevertheless na was hurt because Three was taking Tracy—hurt because na imagined that Three preferred to take Tracy, would find Tracy more fun to be with.

"Don't be so serious, Harp," Three had said, holding the carpenter's chin and laughing. "You're my solemn upright harp, all gold and mournful. We're just going on a one-week trip for the cause." The carpenter had tried to explain that na understood but was still hurt. "You're jealous," Three had said then and laughed gleefully. "Our most serious revolutionary is into possessing nan lover? You want to own me!" The carpenter protested. "I won't tell a soul," Three said, really high now on the joke. "But I knew it. Once a capitalist, always a capitalist!" The carpenter threw out nan arm and pushed Three to the floor. The next morning Three left and neither of them spoke.

For a week the carpenter had thought about nan own seriousness. It was a birth defect, na decided. Na could not help it. Na looked often at nan face in the mirror. Long and stately like a harp. Pale and colorless. Seriousness had found in the movement a camouflage through daily usefulness but now Three, nan lover, was bored with na. Na wanted to have fun. The carpenter pushed away "all work and no play" from childhood and "wet blanket" from adolescence; na held back the past lest it cloud nan mind with a gust of self-pity. Three was right; na was too serious, here, in the present. That was enough to know. But jealous? The carpenter envied Tracy nan carefreeness and was hurt that Three could laugh and go away so easily. Is that jealousy? And possessiveness?

By the time the week was out, the carpenter's feelings of hurt had grown into something else: a huge aching need to hold Three and re-contact, re-mingle, re-involve naself with na totally. Three's absence had sucked out nan insides, leaving a hollow through which nan final jeering words echoed endlessly. Na felt old and dry and finished, doomed to be more serious than ever. Na walked through the week aware of the heaviness of nan step, the literalness of nan every response. The few times that na

108

tried to bring lightness to nan answers, nan own voice sounded like tin. The attempt threw a layer of gloom over nan entire past. By the week's end, na could not remember that na had ever laughed in nan life.

A month before the carpenter had taken a trip with Three to Houston. In the tenuous fog of early morning, they had stopped the car on the highway. An armadillo was on the highway's shoulder, dead. Its crenelated shellback allowed it to survive all enemies except the automobile, so it had lived through the centuries.

Three had never seen an armadillo before; na examined it thoughtfully. "We would have to take off the shell to know it," na said. "Unless the shell *is* knowing it." Three's eyes were crisp against the fog. "The shell is its weapon. To take those hard ridges off its food value would be to give a weapon to its enemy, therefore that hat it wears is a weapon as good as teeth or claws."

"Protection?"

Three insisted. "A weapon itself."

The carpenter shivered. "I would not eat it even if it were shell-less."

"You've never been hungry. But you'd eat it too and salt every mouthful with your tears and cry, 'I have to! I have to!'—to your mind wriggling up on top."

"What are you talking about?" The carpenter put an arm around Three's shoulders and held na close.

"I can't—I just can't believe you won't destroy me," Three turned nan head sideways. "I never cry. I haven't cried since I can remember."

The noise of a car approaching made Three jerk away. "Fuck this system," na shouted. Na slammed the car door and sat stiff inside.

"I'm going for gin," Three said.

The carpenter had longed to hold, stroke, kiss, ignite,

explode, touch Three since dawn. Na had been aware of Three's body inch by inch during the drive, the frustrating meeting, the after-beer. Nan lust was now so heightened it was tapping against nan insides like frantic fingers. Na held on when Three tried to pull away.

"Now now, Harp." Three held the carpenter's face to hold it back. "We can do it just as well with a bottle of gin on the night table. Gin doesn't watch."

"Don't drink."

"I want to." Three pushed suddenly free and smiled in the open door. "I dig walking their Main Street dressed to pass. They think I belong with them. It turns me on."

Na left the door open for the carpenter to come through or shut and pushed the elevator button, practicing a smile in the mirror to go with the shirt (ironed because new), slacks not jeans, regular shoes—a clean, neat, decent smile. The carpenter shut the door.

Twice during the past few weeks the carpenter's orgasm had been interrupted by nan child. One Sunday morning Andy, screaming with a much younger child's pain and terror, had pounded on the door just when all the carpenter's electrical currents were on the brink of descent, effectively terminating everything with a short-circuit flash as the carpenter jumped up in parental response. Andy had smashed nan finger in a window.

A week later, at the safer hour of ten p.m., Andy had run shouting up the stairs and burst through the door when the carpenter was on that same brink, causing the carpenter to flinch and shudder and sit bolt upright like one seized in a nightmare and shout back in terror, "What's the matter?" The police were at the front door, looking for an escaped prisoner who had been locally spotted.

Orgasms, sudden and easy for the carpenter during the early blossoming of passion of a love affair and slower but dependable after the affair was secure,

110

seemed to take a hesitant and difficult vacation during that middle period when the relationship must establish itself. So difficult that na felt na had jumped through nan love-life leaving clusters of paw-prints widely scattered on both sides of the road. A trail of beginnings. And na had returned years later to those few full-fledged lovers (those two) more often and more desperately than na otherwise would have.

Nan affair with Three was in the middle period. Andy's innocent intrusions were resented as fiercely as if they were in fact aggressively planned. This trip to Houston alone with Three in an impregnable hotel room had expanded to proportions of Christmas Eve to a five-year-old, with proportionate dread that the one toy na wanted would not be there.

The carpenter barely allowed Three to mix the drink before na coaxed, kissed, thrust na onto the bed and feverishly made love to na.

Three was not there. Nan body flushed with color and glistened from an obvious orgasm; na spoke love words from somewhere else. The carpenter lay nan wet mouth against a fading shoulder, closing nan eyes. In the beginning, na had had an orgasm naself from giving Three one, as if there were a sensory connection from nan hand or mouth to the brain's sexual trigger. Even now, na almost did. Na lay in that content of almost, waiting for Three to subside. Na pretended Three was present. Na pretended nan touch, a minute later, was not listless. Na pretended na had a second eyelid and closed that, descending into deafness.

The carpenter's responses tentatively came forward, retreated, moved up, back, like a strange animal undecided for too long. The carpenter felt split between being with the animal and with the one luring it; anxiety on both sides was then replaced by impatience on one, increasing the anxiety on the other.

"I am tormenting myself," the carpenter said. Na left the bed to fix a drink. Three was re-dressing in nan Houston clothes when na returned.

111

"Your friends were some help," Three said.

"They're not *my* friends. They . . ."

"You asked them to have a beer after the meeting. You wanted to spend the evening with them."

"Denny asked *us* . . ."

"Denny!" Three wheeled, nan face clenched. "That marble-eyed popcorn-eating pig! If you think that one is into changing anything except nan own bank account you're a fool. And na has the bare-assed nerve to call naself a revolutionary. Dig it. Revolutionary. I'm surprised the word doesn't blister nan tongue. 'You have to use your anger to fight the rich for the poor,' " Three mimicked. "Now let's not get mad at each other oh no honey sugar *sweet*heart . . . I'd like to take that alfalfa and shove it back down nan throat. Your big fat friends aren't going to give us one fucking dime and do you know why? Because of *me*. I'm just too fucking much for them, all that background in the hills. 'My family used to spend the summers in Virginia.' That pig had the nerve to cotton up to me by saying that. Well sugar now that's real nice. Summers in Virginia, huh? I bet you were right near the mill I spent my summers in, and winters and summers and winters. I supported my brothers and if that makes me too coarse for you, tough shit. My old man split and I worked since I was thirteen to feed those kids and I'll be damned if I'm going to listen to anybody tell me about summers in Virginia. I'm glad the old man split, na was as mean as a sick mule but my ma didn't divorce na for all that."

"Listen . . ."

"I don't have to listen. I heard already. My ma didn't have the money to divorce na so na lived every day knowing na could come back and beat us up whenever na felt like it."

"Na could have anyway."

"Fucking correct."

"Drunks can do anything they goddamn please and everybody else . . ."

"I am going to get drunk. On your money."

"Everything is *not* money."

"How would you know? How the fucking hell . . ."

"Shut up. Please, just shut up and get drunk." The carpenter sat on the radiator ledge and stared into a feeder street off Houston's Main. Cars and pedestrians. Four garages on one block. *Jesus Saves. One's A Meal. Liquors.* No other neon.

The plastic glass hit nan back like a slap; the cold gin startled nan skin but not nan mind. Na turned. Three crouched, glaring at the carpenter, nan hands in fists. "Hit me. Go on, hit me."

The carpenter didn't move.

"Or are you too educated to use your fists?"

The carpenter lunged for na and threw na backwards across the bed, the carpenter's knees pinning Three's arms to the mattress. Na sat astride Three, nan hands on nan throat.

"What's the matter with you?" the carpenter shouted. "I love you. What the fucking hell is the matter with you?"

"Strangle me and prove it." Three's eyes were narrow. Na spit, hitting the carpenter's chin.

The carpenter got up and sat in the chair. Three got up and fixed another drink. Na stood in front of the mirror, smoothing the wrinkles on nan new, ironed shirt. The fury of nan face contrasted strangely with the screen of proper dress. Na suddenly saw nan own image: a store-window mannequin shouting revolution.

"Yeah, I have to dress to survive. You don't. That's the fucking privilege you have. You'd look ruling class in a tow sack. They'd kill me in this town if I wasn't wearing their uniform but they can tell by the way you walk and talk who you are. You'd make a first-class revolutionary if you ever did decide to."

"There's not going to be any revolution if you and I can't even discuss money," the carpenter said. "The movement will never . . ."

"Discuss? Let's discuss. Sure. Civilized discuss. Go

113

ahead. You want to discuss. I'm listening."

"Poverty is your throne . . ."

"Fucking correct."

" . . . you think you're the only one who has anything important to say . . ."

"Fucking correct."

" . . . because your background is more real than anyone else's. So you won't even listen to what someone who isn't as poor as you . . ."

"Call Denny." Three stood over the carpenter, eyes flashing. "You want to listen to na, call na. You two can discuss. You want to hear your precious dreams thrown back at you from nan refined mouth, all in words you understand, you just go right ahead. You call it discuss, you discuss the whole fucking night for me. I'm leaving."

Three finished the gin, threw the glass to the floor where it bounded across the green-on-green amoebas of the carpet as the door slammed.

The carpenter stared at the door as na picked up the house telephone and gave a number to the operator. "Denny?" The carpenter's voice was low and urgent and na felt incongruously like a spy. "I'm glad I caught you. Look, don't come tonight. I can't explain now. Look, I'm sorry. I hope you understand."

The carpenter found Three in the second bar na searched. Na stood behind na and spoke to the back of nan ear.

"You're right, about one thing—it scares the shit out of me just to go in these bars looking for you. I love you."

Three didn't turn around. "You'd rather be with Denny in a living room."

"Forget Denny. I love you."

"I don't believe you." Three's voice was empty of any emotion, nan face reflected in the bar's mirror drunk and vulnerable.

The carpenter felt drunk too. Peaceful and detached.

114

"Well, I love you anyway. I'm just going to stand behind you quietly and get drunk with you."

Three suddenly laughed. "If we're going to do that we'd better go back to the hotel room and drink free.

The carpenter concentrated on fitting the key into its complicated slot. Three reached for nan hand and squeezed it painfully hard. "You're the only person in the world I care about. That's why I get so mad at you—I'm afraid you don't love me. You'll leave me." Three was crying.

"Never. I understand you grits," the carpenter said. "I'm from the south too."

Na fixed them both a huge drink as if to get drunk was now a duty. They drank steadily side by side on the bed, repeating that they loved each other, feeling the closeness that accompanies the fact that for this hour at least they were prisoners with each other: neither one could leave this room and go anywhere without being stared at, ridiculed or arrested for drunkenness, neither could talk to another person in the world they were so drunk, only another drunk would do, only the person who had been companion to this point of drunkenness.

"You did think about calling Denny though. Didn't you?"

The carpenter hesitated. "Yes," na said in a near whisper.

"I knew it!"

Before the rage could begin its terrible soar the carpenter grabbed Three's head and held nan face in both hands. "Yes. You're right. I did. Do you see that you're right? Now you have to go to sleep because I can't fight any more."

The carpenter stroked Three's body tough and hard as a corncob, held na until na fell asleep, held na gently after na fell asleep, nan head heavy with sleep, lifeless on the carpenter's shoulder. After such

115

a storm, closeness now was a mixture of hurt anger and love spread apart by a blunt wedge of exhaustion.

The carpenter looked back on that early fight with nostalgia. Recent arguments with Three had involved the cook, and the carpenter felt torn and confused; Three simultaneously identified with the cook, excluding the carpenter from the human race, and viciously attacked na.

"The cook comes from my background, grease and potatoes," Three said. "The only place we fit in is in the kitchen. But the difference between the cook and I is that na'll let you run na and I won't. For you, cook's a tuck-tailed puppy trained to heel. You're probably still in love with na too, you just don't have the guts to admit it because then you'd have to admit you made a mistake with me. I'm one big fucking mistake to you, but then you'd have to admit that your ass made a fool out of those educated brains of yours and your royal pride'll never do that."

In the middle of drilling a hole with the drill-shaft extended, minutes after the cook left, a laugh exploded in the carpenter's mind—laugh expressed in the metaphor of shock. In the course of that argument, Three had shouted another sentence which now reshouted itself in nan absence: "Your past is money and your head is money, and whether you pretend to love me or the cook, we're small change as far as you're concerned."

The carpenter had not heard "small change" as a pun and nan laugh now was relief. Na could deal with intellectual shock. Na could analyse. Na could divide nan brain into teams and contest the truth of anything.

Na could conclude.

Money is a synonym for value; Three does not feel that I love na; Three is jealous of the cook because na

116

thinks na is the same person as the cook, indistinguishable to a lover. When specie is wanted all banks are equal.

Three is jealous; I compare. Tracy has wit and joy and the kind of chemical rhythm which spins one's own mood faster and I envy and covet nan qualities. I compare myself to Tracy and come out bland and pale. Wherein then am I special? I have believed all my life in my specialness, fostered by two grandmothers. If my specialness disappears because Three prefers Tracy . . . I am suffering from a wound to my specialness. How dare Three not recognize . . .? If I have to metamorphose myself into someone nearer to Tracy I will have to start from way behind.

Na turned back on the drill and drove it through— a perfect hole. Na took the next two by four and made another. A third. Holes straight and clean as a thought. The drill was more than a machine; it was master of the exact transformation of the idea of hole into hole.

I should have gone to Houston after work last night and thrust myself into Three's presence in the open after-midnight hours to seize and shake and claim na as my lover. (Imagination offered up the thrill Three would experience, cast as most highly desired treasure—escaping gold.) You belong to me, I would have shouted, my force sucking out nan doubts, my act declaring proof of nan value, my demand attesting nan worth to all the world. To Three naself, also.

To Three naself, also?

The carpenter concluded that Three was wrong; Three was jealous; the carpenter naself was far from jealous, felt in fact no emotion at all that was anywhere near the one commonly called jealousy.

No emotion. The drill rested; gleamingly inert, its former whirling vibrated echoes in the carpenter's mind. Na felt fragile and explosive. Na probed nervously: why don't I go back to that safer love-affair? Why did I so easily accept the cook's rejection of me

117

in favor of the children and so doggedly force myself to understand Three's insults? Understand. I am a goddamn parent to the corners of my soul.

The cook was my best friend and I was in love with na too, wasn't I? We were as happy as children enriching our world with sex. Na remembered the gentleness of nan first night with the cook; tenderness re-experienced flushed nan blood. Na balanced on the edge of that night. Na thought na could tell Three . . .

Thinking that name so vividly evoked the person that the carpenter spoke out loud, "Three." Gentleness collapsed like a ping-pong ball rocking in boiling water, puffed artificially huge and too thin. The force of nan love for Three overwhelmed confusion and memory, na smelled nan presence in nan mind, nan whole body throbbed with the sudden inrush of Three in that thought-produced vacuum. Na was as swollen now with urgency as na had been bloated earlier with defense. Na cried out nan name again, "Three;" nan voice was thin with the pain of seeing Three as a person totally separate of the first time.

Chris opened the door, letting in a pale rectangle of sun. The carpenter turned on the drill briefly, to dispel the irritation na felt at the interruption.

"I'm sorry to interrupt you," Chris said. "It's sort of important." Nan face was startingly beautiful. Aristocratic? Serious and classless. "I want to move into town, live with someone I know . . .na is called Duffy and works at the Gulf station."

"Live with?"

The expression in Chris's eyes clarified the ambiguity: *live* with.

"But I thought you and Leslie . . .?"

"We *were*. Leslie feels na should be with blacks now. But this thing with Duffy is different. I mean Leslie and I were best friends—it was so safe, like being wrapped inside a pillow with a mirror . . ."

118

"*Safe?*"

"Finally, safe. We understood each other and supported each other which pulled out all my anger. I thought you'd understand." The carpenter thought na heard the echo of an earlier whine through Chris's flat explanatory patience. "It was the same thing as you and the cook—you know, internal, a sinking back into last week. You left the cook for Three, didn't you? You could have stayed in the pillow. With Three, you have to reach up. At least I assume that was the reason; I guess I don't really know."

"Yeah." The word was noncommittal, a stall.

"But with Duffy . . .I've never met anyone like Duffy before in my whole life. Na is completely different from me—we don't even mean the same things by the same words!" Chris's grey eyes were bare of caution.

The carpenter suddenly laughed. "You're baring your eyes! Can you do that—like teeth?"

"I feel so alive!" Chris said, hugging nan parent. "I knew you'd understand." Just as Chris left, na said with a chilling lilt to nan voice, "It's what you said about chaos, isn't it?"

When Three returned that night, the carpenter took nan hand and pulled na to the side of the house, to the perfectly-sanded porch.

"Listen. You don't have to be jealous of the cook, of anyone. I am wholly committed to you," the carpenter said, nan eyes glowing with seriousness.

"Never?"

"Never."

"Since when?"

"This minute. We'll never fight again, I'll never fight you again. I promise."

Three laughed and held the carpenter very close. "We'll fight again, my perfect harp. Because we

119

love each other."

"We love us."

"I missed you," Three said. "But I thought and I learned something: mainly I'm afraid that loving you is going to fuck up my head."

"Your head's in this too."

"Wait a minute. I'm not going to change for you."

"Yes, you are. You're going to change and so am I."

12

Excerpts from meetings: January-February

"Why don't we ask the city council to let us use the building?"

"And smile? Ask nicely and say please?"

"I know nobody here *wants* to ask. We'd all rather take. But if it's a way of getting the building . . ."

"Bullshit. Until we learn how to say, You on that throne, you *got* no power because we didn't give you any by *asking* you for this—until we say that by our actions we're still in first grade."

"They wouldn't give it to us. I've been to every open meeting the council and the school board have held and every issue like this gets the same vote: two to one against. That's the spread. To bring it up, to ask, would polarize them right off and make them determined not to give it to us. So then if we refuse to accept their negative and take the building anyway, they would treat us like disobedient children who had to be spanked on principle. They could never give us a building after they said "no." I know them. They would feel they were condoning insurrection. Our only hope is that the town or someone with influence or press opinion will sway their thinking after we've taken it and they will find it easier to let us keep it."

"Do you think that will happen?"

"No. I just think it's the only chance we've got."

"Once we have a building and set everything up, what are we going to do about people from town say who want to work with us? They may have other ideas about how things should be run."

"They may outnumber us."

"Wouldn't that be outasight!"

"We'll have to maintain control . . ."

"We'll have to, but we'll be accused of it too."

"Okay. But once we get it started the way we know it should be, we can't let people come in and turn it back into the same old social services center."

"What's the problem? Whoever works decides. That'll take care of itself once we get going."

"I think we should set it up now. You know what happened in New York, at Fifth Street. No one was in charge and there was chaos, and when there's chaos people start shouting 'elitism,' partly because they feel frantic."

"I thought the trouble with Fifth Street was that it succeeded. No one could believe it. So people sort of brought it down to prove they were right in the first place for not believing in it."

"I never thought of that."

"Nothing was wrong with Fifth Street. It was so beautiful everyone fell in love. *That's* what happened."

The cook brought five leaflets to the meeting, each one written in English on one side, Spanish on the other. Na held up the first one and read the words: To touch, to relate, to break down barriers between ourselves, to act . . .

"*Barriers* is spelled wrong," Meredith said. "You have it: b-a-r-r-i-*a*-r-s and it should be, *e*-r-s."

"I thought it looked funny," the cook said. "I guess we can change it."

"Leave it," Three said. "So we can't spell."

"Change it," Leslie said and laughed. "You saw that IQ test they did on the black and white children. Honey, even *we* can spell."

"Wait a minute," Stubby said. Na stood up. "There are how many thousand people in this town who need to be reached, they're out there waiting for us to get them involved, and you start right off with the one thing that's going to turn them off: *touch*. We have to reach these people on the basis of the real problems in their lives, like jobs and child care, and you make it sound as if we're establishing a hip orgy where everyone sits around *touching*. We're dealing with a puritan culture and to these people *touch* is a dirty word. You can't influence them . . ."

"You're insulting them," Leslie said. "You're treating them like a mass of numbers we have to 'influence'—like we need that figure to add to our publicity report. People know who loves them and your kind of talk doesn't make me feel you love anybody."

"Love them? I know them," Stubby said. "And believe me we're not going to get to first base if we don't cut out this talk about 'touch' and 'relate' and get down to the real issues which are money and class privilege. That is loving them."

"Now you talk like you mean 'love' but don't *love*," Leslie said.

"I'm just telling you what will turn people off . . ."

"I don't believe that. I think I turn you off."

"Now let's not get into a personal argument," Stubby said.

Leslie stood up. "It is personal." Nan voice was low

and clear. "Every time you open your mouth you talk about the people this and the people that and I been sitting here for six months listening to that and I know I'm a person and I'm black and I'm one of your homosexuals the 'people' can't deal with and every time you open your mouth you make me feel like I don't exist, like I'm invisible as far as you're concerned and you want to keep it that way. Well, that's some revolution. Big deal. I'm invisible in the old system and I'm going to get to be invisible in the new. Well, you can just take that kind of revolution and shove it up your ass or in your belly button or back in your mouth, for me. I'm not sticking around here to be your token black for the newspapers as long as I 'behave' myself. I know one thing for sure—I may not belong out there but I sure don't belong in here either." Leslie was at the door when Chris caught na and went out with na. The people by the door followed them; then the rest of the group except Stubby.

Stubby sat down among the empty chairs; Sweeper turned back, came and sat next to na.

"Now I'm going to say something," Sweeper said. "I think some of us . . . you . . . I know *I'm* just plain scared to death to go and set up a center for homosexuals in this town—even if it is only one out of all the projects. I have nightmares that they're going to tar-and-feather me, drag me naked behind a horse, cut open my belly and fill it with ants. Now you can say that my imagination is running away with me, but I mean it, I'm flat scared stiff. Every time I think about it I want to run away—I mean that. I'm ready to leave town half the time. Now if someone could just promise me that I'm crazy . . . I even wish someone would laugh at me . . ."

"I am not scared!" Stubby shouted.

13

March 3 was Texas Independence Day. They planned to take over the building the following Saturday night.

The building chosen was the old elementary school in their neighborhood. The residential section of the town had grown the other way and only businesses and a few old people's rooming houses were still in this area. An adjacent section though was a community of low-income people, occupying houses built over twenty years before on the GI bill. The original owners had moved out and the houses were rented to young families or single people. There had been a new elementary school built when the GI houses came and both schools were filled to capacity during the fifties; beginning in the sixties, the old one no longer served its immediate neighborhood, an annex was built onto the new school and with the depression of 1962, the old school was abandoned.

125

The group chose it partly because it belonged to the people of the neighborhood and partly because it was beautiful. Built one story only, of wood originally painted white, it rambled across a half-block of over-grown playgrounds. It was a low structure, scaled to the size of its pupils, with windows and doors in every possible space for pre-air-conditioning ventilation and easy exit. A columned arcade ran along two sides to shield the pupils from the excessive Texas sun. Mature live-oak and Chinese tallow trees, huge now, dwarfed the thing they sheltered. By March 1, teased by a week of tropical weather, hundreds of branches of forsythia had opened into lemon-yellow blossoms, spraying the playgrounds with sunshine in shade.

"The electricity works. It's still on," the reconnaissance group reported. They had entered the building one morning equipped with a ventilated box and a butterfly net in case they were questioned. No one had noticed them at all.

"There isn't an intact window in the place. Every inch of floor space is covered with glass—and leaves and whiskey bottles and junk."

"The windows don't matter in weather like this."

"But the plumbing has been ripped out. Pulled out of the wall, broken off, smashed with an ax. It looks like it was done deliberately, but it may have been vandalism. There isn't any water at all."

"If you weren't such an aristocrat to begin with," Three said to the carpenter. "You would have seen that you should have become a plumber instead of a carpenter."

"But wait until you see the kitchen. It's huge—big walk-in refrigerators and an enormous stove, all in perfect condition. We could feed the whole town."

"All we have to do is hook up the gas."

"All?"

"We'll take food for a few days anyway."

"What'll we do for toilets?"

"Use kitty litter," Nicky said.

126

"Perfect!"

"I read that somewhere. You get a plastic garbage can and a liner and put in kitty litter and lysol. It's like a portable toilet, see. It's the same thing."

"We also need some plastic for the windows."

"Yeah. I guess it could rain."

"It could do worse than that. There's a norther forecast for the weekend."

"We're going to take the truck and buy supplies. What else?"

"A real norther?"

"It's supposed to go down to ten degrees."

"Ten degrees? That sky is bluer than August."

"What are we going to do for heat?"

"We could wait a month."

"There's a gasoline heater where Chris works. Maybe Duffy could borrow it."

"Did Chris tell Duffy about this?" Three said.

"You know na did. They're lovers," the carpenter said.

"I didn't think anyone but us was supposed to know."

"Who is Duffy?"

"Nan parent is on the police force," Meredith said. "Great."

"Is Duffy against it—taking over the school, I mean."

"No. I don't think so," the carpenter said. "Na doesn't understand why we don't ask the city council if we can have the building, but na isn't . . ."

"Neither do I," Meredith said.

"Come on, we're going shopping. Where's the fucking list?"

"Somebody listen to this press release and see if I've got it right," Tracy said. " 'Pursuant to our negotiations with the city council . . .' "

"Pursuant? What does that mean?"

"Well, actually, it means 'following'—in the sense of it's yet to come, but it sounds like it means 'following' in the other sense. I mean I wanted them to think we were already negotiating."

"Brilliant."

"Does it really?"

"Got any more words like that?"

"Let me read the rest. ' . . . we of the neighborhood of the Shadyside Elementary School . . .' "

" 'Former.' "

"Yeah, that's important."

" . . . former Shadyside Elementary School which was abandoned by this town ten years ago are reclaiming our school for our use. It is a crime against the people of this town that buildings built by our money are left idle, haven for robbers, muggers, rapists and other undesirables . . .' "

"What about 'hiding place?' 'Haven' sounds too poetic."

"Okay. ' . . . other undesirables and a constant reminder to the people of this neighborhood that our property is so lightly regarded that the city council does not even bother to protect or maintain it."

"That's good. Hit them on the property angle."

"It's true."

"We didn't pay to have that school built."

"No, but the people we're speaking for did."

"Go on."

" 'Therefore we are occupying this school . . . no, have occupied this abandoned school building in order to set up services which this neighborhood needs, for the people of this community: health care, child care, a food co-op, classes in self-defense, plumbing and e-lectricity, a people's theater, a twenty-four hour shelter, a crisis center for children, teenagers, old people, marriage failures and communication splits of all kinds, and a center for homosexuals."

"Why did you put the homosexual center last?"

"Well, I didn't want to seem to be burying it in the middle."

"It doesn't matter. That's the first thing they're going to pick up."

128

"I think it's very good. Don't you want to say something about—'since the town has failed to provide for the needs of the people we have no other choice but to provide for our own?'"

"How could anyone disagree with that? It's the American tradition of self-help."

"You'll see."

"Okay, it's going out to the Evening Star, the Texas Observer in Austin, Pacifica and both Houston papers, the local radio station . . ."

"That's the same as the Evening Star. They're both owned by J. C. 'Jim' Smith."

"They each get one anyway. And the members of the city council and the mayor. Stubby's going to send one to the Spanish paper even though it won't come out until the next week."

"What about television?"

"That'll have to come from Houston."

"I know someone at Channel 13."

"They won't come all the way down here."

"Well, send them one anyway."

"That's very good, Tracy."

"I'll have to telephone them in from a pay phone downtown after the rest of you start out. It'll cost a fortune in change."

"Use the phone at Chris's Gulf Station. They're open until midnight on Saturdays and no one is there except Chris and Duffy."

"They lock up the change at seven o'clock though. Someone has to go to the bank this afternoon."

"Have you seen Stubby?" Meredith said. "We have a play for Sunday afternoon and we need to know some Spanish."

"I haven't seen na since the meeting when Leslie left," Carter said. "But then I haven't wanted to."

"Na hasn't been here," Andy said.

"Na hasn't slept here?" Three asked.

"Not last night." Andy was sure; na had checked nan room at midnight and at five this morning, with Nicky.

"Nicky and I are spies."

By ten o'clock that night everyone was assembled in the living room with sleeping bags, canteens, flashlights and musical instruments. The truck was packed with food, plastic for the windows, equipment for the home-made toilets, a space heater, electric heaters, light bulbs, tools of all kinds. Stubby was still absent and the temperature had dropped to nine degrees. Sleet plinked against the windows on the north; wind scratched through the walls of the house. Carter was plucking nan guitar while two conversations were going around the room: Shouldn't we choose another night because of the weather? and, Where is Stubby?

The weather was seen by some as an omen, a warning which commented ominously on Stubby's absence: Had Stubby gone to the police? Had na been a spy all along?

"That would sure explain nan piss-ass puss," Nicky said.

"Na *is* a spy," Andy said. Nan face was twinkling with anger. "I knew it!"

"Suppose na is?" the cook said to the carpenter.

"Then tonight we either take over a building or we expose a pig," the carpenter said and grinned. "Either way we win."

"If na is . . ." the cook said. "No, Stubby's too obvious. Aren't spies supposed to blend in?"

Stubby arrived at ten-thirty. "I want to explain," na began, standing in front of the door, nan eyes moving from face to face. "Hold your questions a minute. Quiet a minute. Now listen. I've been thinking since the last meeting . . . I'm not going to go into the building with you people. In the first place, I'm opposed to this action as everyone knows, and it will be hard enough for the rest of you without having me along dragging you down—even if I say nothing, everyone knows how I feel. But in the second place, I've concluded that I'm just not going to do something I don't

130

believe in. Having made that decision, I think it's the right decision. And there is a personal reason which I can't divulge now. No, not now. I'll tell you tomorrow or the next day. Well, I can't and I'm not going to. So I'll do what I can from the outside—I'll help Tracy send out the press releases and then come back here . . ." Stubby's face was flushed and nan hands were shaking; na stared at the floor. "Or I'll just go away if you want me to. But if I can help, by staying outside as a liaison, then I'd like to do that."

14

The former Shadyside Elementary School was ten blocks away. Sleet had turned to hail by the time they had walked three of them. There were tiny pellets of ice bouncing across the black asphalt like crystal beads, hitting the shining wet black surface of the road so rapidly that to the eye the road became water and the drops rain and then the road solid and the drops hail, and back again. Several people held out their hands and collected the ice pellets and stared at the road and said, "Hail," out loud.

There were about twenty-five of them bunched into a quarter block. Everyone was so thoroughly dressed that only faces glowed in the passing street lights, each so alive that a closest friend felt a rush of excitement at seeing the most familiar face suddenly new.

As they turned a corner, a new figure came running up to the group, hair frozen in white strings; na began to overtake the others, peering backwards into each face. Toward the front of the line, na entered and put an arm around another.

"Leslie," Chris said, holding nan shoulder. "I had to come too."

Leslie grinned. "I knew you would."

They entered the building through a window, one by one but so swiftly they looked as if they had practiced. They entered so smoothly, without a head bump or single trip, they appeared to be performing a perfectly-rehearsed dance. Each watched even as na was an acting part and saw that they were as together as a well-planned machine. Twenty-six times a figure stepped over the window sill, balanced, and landed inside without breaking the rhythm of the music one imagined were accompanying this movie reality.

They stared. The room was a space enclosed and strange, a house whose history or builder no longer mattered; theirs.

The sheets of plastic had been stapled to the windows, the floor was swept, Carter was playing "The Old Grey Mare" on the guitar and the cook was dancing around the rice-pot when they heard the brief siren out front.

The carpenter had been delegated to deal with the police. Na straightened nan expression to grey seriousness and stood tall in the doorway. Na addressed the police as "officer."

Na explained. They were negotiating with the mayor and the city council; the community wanted to rehabilitate this building and use it to serve the needs of the community: child care, mobile health services, education—its original purpose.

The older policeperson was the same age as the carpenter, the same height; they each spoke in a voice near enough the same for the officer to recognize the accent.

The police looked around. The older one saw the children and food and guitar and smiled. The younger

133

stared at Leslie and pointed out the space heater. The carpenter quickly described its BTU's, its area efficiency, its gallon capacity. The older was satisfied that there was no danger from fire and prepared to leave. The younger scowled and followed.

Five minutes later, "The Old Grey Mare" cast out the freezing cold and diminished the sound of sleet against plastic to a background plink.

"I'm too old to cut up like this," the carpenter said the next morning. Nan eyes were red and nan bones ached at every joint.

"Pacifica's here. They want to know who our leader is."

"It's freezing outside. Shut the door."

"I'm doing a lot of fetching and carrying," the cook said, handing the carpenter a fifth cup of coffee.

"Who wants to speak for Pacifica's tape?"

"Me, but I'm scared."

"Two of you do it together."

"This has got to be the world's greatest Sunday morning!"

"You tell 'em, Sweeper."

"Me? I'll lose my kids."

"They can't identify your voice from a tape."

"Shut the door!"

"My god, it's the resource redistributor!"

Grinning above two sacks of groceries, Dallas found the carpenter and Carter and stood in front of them waiting to be hugged.

"I've been wanting to come back and see you all and then I heard this on the radio this morning," Dallas said. "I let out a yell right there in the Piggley-Wiggley and bought everything I could carry. You did it! Boy, have you got this town buzzing. Everybody on the bus was talking about it, half of 'em for you and half of 'em shocked outa their drawers. Do something with this food so I can get away from that microphone."

134

"What are they saying?" the carpenter asked.

"That they're going to set rangers on the borders of Texas three feet apart and keep those dirty communist queers out of our home. A homosexual center in this town. They ignored the rest of the projects. Boy, you sure did it. The people on the bus were moving all over the place. Them that's for you would get up and move away from them that's against you, and sit by someone else who'd get up and move away from them. I never saw so much moving around on one bus in my life. They were shifting all over like they had the measles and calling each other by those terrible first names they use when they're trying to control their fists." Dallas patted nan pocket. "Who do I give the bail money to?"

Last night's ice storm, the worst since 1951, was blamed for an additional disaster: the town's newest office building had blown up early this morning. Several gas pilot lights had gone out in the building's basement when gas pressure dropped in response to a freezing citizenry's thermostats turned to maximum; later the gas pressure returned, gas filling the basement. Somewhere a loyal pilot light remained; when the gas reached it, it exploded. That was the fire department's theory. They were all downtown, along with the Sunday police force, to keep the townspeople safe from their entertainment.

"The cops are torn in two," Dallas said. "Do they get to watch the fire or do they get to come after you? There's gonna be eighteen cops signing up for Sunday duty tomorrow."

Bells rang out the end of the church service a block away; in a few minutes the elderly entered the schoolhouse in a wave of pastel and grey.

"You remembered the old folks," one said, patting the cook's arm. "Bless your hearts, you thought about the old folks."

"Young people don't want their hearts blessed," nan companion said. "I declare, that's a sweet child." Nan

135

fingers, fingering everything in sight from the habit of no longer trusting sight alone, had reached Nicky's uncombed hair.

"Fuck that," Nicky said, slapping nan hand away. Na slapped Nicky's back. Nicky slapped. Na slapped again. The cook stepped between them.

"Will you have bingo?" na said to the cook. "There's no need; the church does that. There's not much you can do, you'll find."

"Not much? There's everything," the first one said, shaking nan finger like a skinny pencil at nan companion's face. "Some of us still have ideas left, you know."

"Come along, cousin. We'll come back next month when it's warm—if they're still here. Any ideas you got are bound to be so new it won't hurt to sit on them."

"Bless your hearts," the first one said over nan shoulder.

From another church, on the other side of town, a car drove up. One of the visitors was from the black newspaper.

"We didn't know there was a black newspaper here," Tracy said, handing them a copy of the press release.

"We didn't know you all were here until today," the reporter said.

"You really took this here schoolhouse for the people?"

"We sure did."

"Well, I just had to come and see for myself. Couldn't believe it when I heard it on the radio. For us! You're too much."

"We would of brought you some beer except it's not one o'clock yet. Wouldn't do to be breaking the law, now would it?" The youngest grinned and slapped Tracy's arm. "Y'all are something else."

"Look at the way they've got this place decorated, Vee." Na pointed at the wall and read aloud, " 'Our

136

love is changing the world.' That's real nice."

"We passed them on our way over here," the reporter said. "They're sending the sheriff. Cops must be busy at the fire."

"Now?"

"The sheriff is coming now?"

"They were gathering when we passed." The reporter took out a notebook. "How many are you? You got kids here too?"

"We're leaving now, Vee," nan companion said. "I've been that route before." Na looked around the room again. "This room sure makes me feel good. Maybe you better come out and sit in the car with us," na said to Leslie. "Come on, baby. You're too young for them deputies to mess with."

"I'm staying," Leslie said.

"We got to go *now*, sugar."

The room grew silent as the siren sounded and rapidly drew closer. Everyone in the room stood as tall and straight as possible, listening without a word.

The reporter stood still; the other visitors walked quickly to the front door. The youngest turned at the door. "They ain't just whistlin' Dixie," na said to Leslie. "Come on, child."

"Go, Leslie." The carpenter heard nan own voice shake.

Leslie stared at the group in the door with sudden fear. "Stop scaring me," na said then, grinning.

The visitors disappeared. Dallas, with nan usual facility, had vanished without anyone seeing na go. The children edged closer to their parents. The carpenter stood at the front door, waiting for the sheriff.

"Move aside," the sheriff said, entering the room with half a dozen deputies following. "All right. The game's over. Get those kids out before they're hurt. The rest of you are under arrest."

"Press," the black reporter said, showing nan card.

"Nigger press," the sheriff said. "Law says press has to

137

be back twenty feet when arrests are being made and this room is being arrested. Now get on the sidewalk and stay clear."

"There is no such law," the carpenter said. "The press is here to witness . . ."

Suddenly the carpenter saw the familiar face of the one called Tiny, the one they had tied up at the carnival in the fall. The carpenter felt a wash of adrenalin draw na as alert as a mouse.

"That's the leader. Get that one." Tiny pointed to the carpenter and at the same time raised the other arm and swung at the carpenter's face with an iron pipe. The carpenter dodged and caught the pipe in nan hand just before it would have cracked the cook's head. Tiny's fist landed in the carpenter's kidneys and nan knees buckled to the floor.

"Settle down, Tiny," the sheriff said mechanically. "We can handle it." And over nan shoulder, "Okay, now get these dirty reds out of here!"

Sweeper felt rage from a lifetime turn nan face purple and nan eyes dark as knives. Na drew back nan foot, kicked as hard as na could, aiming for the sheriff's genitals. Na hit nan shins. Instantly, a gun butt came down on Sweeper's skull with a thwamp. Sweeper fell into a fat lump.

Four deputies picked na up and dragged na spread-eagled to the waiting car, the sheriff tapping nan gun like a stick against Sweeper's crotch.

Three wedged a knee into Tiny's leg and threw na onto the floor; Three grabbed for the hand that still held the iron pipe and felt the thumb joint crack before na was caught by a deputy, nan own arm twisted up nan back. Three bit the deputy's hand as hard as na could.

"Goddamn perverts," the deputy said, slapping Three's ear into ringing deafness.

Leslie's voice came out in a strange high singsong: "You're big and white, brave and white, smart as the white of a hardboiled egg and right as the white of the stripe of the flag . . . you're tall and white, bright and white, strong as the white of a tub of lard . . . you honor the white, salute . . ."

"Shut that nigger up!"

A hand covered Leslie's nose and mouth, pushing into nan face; one deputy easily dragged na to the car; another followed by the side, whacking Leslie's body wherever nan stick could land.

"Which one's the leader?" the captain asked.

"They won't say."

"Search 'em and book 'em."

They were taken separately into small cells of concrete so old and damp they looked and smelled like urinals. Three was first.

"Take off your shoes and shake out your socks," the policewoman said.

"You take them off."

The policewoman called the sergeant.

"She doesn't want to take my socks off," Three said. "She is afraid they stink. Maybe they do, but my politics don't."

The sergeant pushed Three to the floor and, with his foot on her back, told the policewoman to take off her shoes, pull down her pants, spread her cheeks.

The sergeant pushed his foot into Three's buttocks before removing it. "Now you so smart you know you don't have to put them clothes back on neither if you think it's gonna incriminate you," he said.

"Cops are real tall when they're standing on a woman," Three said.

Inside the jail, the men of the world were represented by those present—from the sergeant's open hatred to the muffled curiosity of a citizen bystander. As they answered official questions, they were aware of the trivial nature of their own differences: whereas previously they had all felt that their group of women, coming together from different spheres, lives, ages,

139

had meant that any conclusion the group reached had the validity of convergence, now—the thought was a glare from the flatface opposite—they appeared as a collection of one minute sub-genre of strangeness coincidentally gathered into a tiny room. They were no more than a single gritty-eyed headache in the life of a giant.

They were joined to each other like petals of a five-pointed flower, dependent upon the joining for any life at all. An extreme consciousness of physical self was the center of their flower, awareness of individual body outlines which exagerrated the previous absence of such a separation into forms of flesh. Each one was conscious of her own and the other four soft and oddly-shaped bodies badly dressed in familiar clothes, suddenly shabby and bizarre. Each heard her own voice chant of a shared childhood, drumming against chambers built to house expensive responsibility. Every damp work-shoe sat identically flat on the concrete floor.

The space they had created (up until now) for themselves had formed a vacuum wherein they could scatter and diverge, where shape was unnecessary; a totally safe, conflictless space within which all tensions, attacks, storms were between/among their own members. Now they were herded down a corridor by the policewoman and felt they had been suddenly bunched like iron filings by a magnet. A second ago, unity had seemed a concentration, force for change; now—it was the contrast that was sharpest—they thought they had been rolled into one ball in order to be stamped out by one efficient foot.

"But you're our sister," Chris said to the policewoman. "You're one of us."

The policewoman's smile automatically accepted inclusion but her eyes were wary and refusing. "Are you all from around here?" she asked Chris, locking the door with a ladylike click.

140

"We live here," Chris said. "We took over an aban . . ."

"I don't know what you did," the policewoman said, and her shoes clicked off the steps out of sight.

For now, they locked their hearts into each other and felt love like the force of the poles.

Their cell measured about six by six. There was a shelf across the back, bench height; a seatless toilet at one end. Daylight came through a high window opposite.

"Now this is real nice for an old jail," Three said. Chris and Leslie sat solemnly on the bench. "Let's sing 'Deep in the Heart of Texas' for them." Three played an imaginary guitar and clapped vigorously between stanzas.

"Cut out the noise, girls." The policewoman appeared at the bars.

"Look, you're our sister, too," the carpenter said.

"We just want to sing," Three said.

"No clapping."

"All right," the carpenter said. "I'll sing. Please try to refrain from applauding. It won't be hard since I can't sing. Is anyone here old enough for 'Remember Pearl Harbor and Remember the Alamo?' Cook's not here, fortunately for her, not for you." The carpenter sang four lines of World War II patriotism in a scratchy, sonorous voice. "I also know, 'Oh beautiful beautiful Texas' " . . . she sang . . . " 'The most beautiful land that I know/ The land where our forefathers/ Fought in the Alamo . . . You can live on the plains or the prairie/ Or down where the sea breezes blow/ And still be in beautiful Texas/ The most beautiful land I know!" Leslie smiled which made the carpenter do a dance of awkward appreciation. "Now, everybody: 'The eyes of Texas are upon you/ All the livelong day/ The eyes of Texas are upon you/ You can not get away . . .' " The last phrase was shouted.

The policewoman reappeared. "That's enough, girls. Cut out the noise."

"We wouldn't let them call you a police girl," the carpenter said.

"If you don't quiet down I'll have to separate you," the policewoman said.

"We all came out of a policewoman. That's what a mother is. You have to make us behave so the men can get on with their big work . . ."

"Our dossiers," Three said.

The policewoman tried to smile; backed away. "I'm just following orders."

"I'm cold," Sweeper said.

"You've got a lump on your head the size of a persimmon," Three said, feeling it. "Pretend it's summer. We're having a pignic. We're roasting fat sausages on shotguns and for dessert we'll toast those soft white marshmallows they have for brains. Come on, Harp, get that fire going. Sweeper's cold. This really tastes funny for a potato chip." Three reached to her chewing mouth and stared at air caught in her fingers. "No wonder. It's all bristles."

"Must be a slice of life," the carpenter said.

"Here, Harp, have a bite of this here pig tongue," Three said.

"Too dirty."

"How could it be dirty? It came from the general's own commissary. Let me smell it. Pugh. That's rank, child."

"Did you see that menu posted where we came in? I'm awfully hot in this coat," the carpenter said, taking it off and tucking it around Sweeper. " 'Cunt dinner,' it said. 'Hot tits and dark meat tomorrow.' "

"That's law and order down here," Three said. "Lay down the law and order women to lay down."

"They sure are afraid of elementary education," the carpenter said. " 'Tiny Jack Horner sat in a corner . . .' A horner is someone who makes horns, you know. A cuckold. 'Stuck in his thumb . . .' "

"I wish I'd gotten his third thumb," Three said. "I heard the bone break with my own ears. While I still

142

had two good ears."

"Sweeper ought to lie down. Leslie too."

"We all should. Everybody put on a good show this afternoon. The sheriff especially got a real kick out of Sweeper."

"The only way we can all lie down is on the floor. We're lucky we have our coats because the floor is filthy."

"If we all lie down together we might have to touch each other and that's even filthier, isn't it? Somebody help me," Three said. "I can't make Leslie laugh."

"Let's be practical," the carpenter said. "We ought to lie with our feet to the bars in case their night sticks are in the mood for music later. We wouldn't want our heads over there being tempting. We all know how we tempt."

"We'll have to put our heads under the bench then," Three said. "Do you think we can breathe under there?"

"Maybe if we put on airs."

"No, that one missed, Harp," Three said. "You're trying too hard."

"I am. Actually, I didn't want to say it but there might be mice under there."

"You just brought up my favorite subject," Three said. "Do you know what my theory is . . . that a mouse is really a soft silky cunt and that's why all the writers and culture makers show ladies terrified of a mouse running up their legs. Because that's the way culture-makers define 'lady,' hoping to make it true. No, I'm not kidding. Every now and then there's a fable—like the mouse that chewed away the net that held the lion—and that's how we know what a mouse is and how much power it could have. The first Freud wrote that thing about the farmer's wife, and those mice were blind to boot. We've been brainwashed with these mouse stories and it's all part of the same old plot. Even Eldridge Cleaver couldn't improve on the line: What are you, a man or a mouse? You know a

143

black eye is called a 'mouse' and a moustache is called a 'mouse'—that's for visual resemblance. And to call a place a mousetrap is no compliment—that's always the proof of what any word really means: if it's an insult, it refers to us. I've thought about this a lot. I'm sure it's true. The last thing we should be afraid of is mice. Now a rat, that's a different animal."

"What about the mouse that roared?"

"Makes everybody laugh. Ridiculous idea." Three sat down on the floor and put her chin on her knees. "So if we all sit here as quiet as . . ."

The policewoman stood on her side of the bars. "All right, get up, you. You can't sit on the floor."

"Why not?"

"Sit on the bench, ladies," she said. "You can't sit on the floor."

Three slowly got up.

"Might be mice around," the policewoman said and left.

The carpenter reached out her arm to encircle Three's shoulders. "Watch it," Three said, pushing the arm away. "You think they allow love in here? What are we going to do for dinner? I'm sick of pork. The Jews are right. Too dirty. Hey, guard! Bring us a menu, we've been sitting here for hours."

They had been in jail for only two hours when a man came through sweeping; he came into their cell with a broom and the carpenter felt a chilling impulse, from a surge of envy at his privileged activity, to grab the broom away from him and sweep sweep sweep.

"The worst of this is that we can't even run for our lives," the carpenter said. "In case of fire or flood, we're dependent upon someone remembering that we're here and humanely releasing us. Is it going to depress anyone if I share my philosophical conclusions with you—this is the first time I've ever been in jail. The essential thing about being able to run for your life is that then you can sit in

144

a tree later and work out whether your move was cowardly or intelligent. If you don't get the choice you don't get to decide, your brain atrophies, your body slides passively to the floor, you probably melt. So it's important to decide about little things. Shall I have a drink of water? Shall I now? Shall I wait? Who else would like a drink of water? I have a mint. Who will have a mint. I think we are in English class. Chris, I . . ."

"Just leave me alone, Mom."

Dinner came at four—two cheese sandwiches apiece, made with one slice of raisin bread, one of white; tepid tea with sugar. Three began eating, looked around, saw that no one else was.

"Eat it, we're paying for it," she said. "In fact, I bet this sandwich is going to cost us more per vitamin . . ."

"Vitamin where?"

"See that raisin? You know what a hero is? A hunk of beef between two women. I'm bored, Harp."

"Shh, Leslie's asleep," Chris said.

"Eat your supper, Chris," the carpenter said.

"It was your mother's singing got it for us," Three said. "Sweeper, you better eat too. It'll warm you up. This bread takes a lot of chewing."

"Those are the dirtiest, rottenest, ugliest, meanest . . ." Sweeper's rage suddenly returned and her face was clenched as if the sheriff were once again in front of her foot. "I don't know what to call them. That sheriff is the sorriest excuse for a human being that ever drew breath. I know one thing for sure: the minute I get out of here I'm going to take . . ."

"A bath in a room without walls like these," Three said. "These are listening walls."

"I don't care if they all hear me. I'll say it again any day of the week. I went to school with that big oaf that came in there with an iron pipe and nobody in his right mind would make him a deputy.

145

The whole town knows he is a can of garbage. I was just getting ready to tell the sheriff that that beast had slipped in when the sheriff says, 'Settle down, Tiny.' Like he was talking to a glass of alka-seltzer. Well, if the sheriff thinks he can make deputies out of lame-brains he can't control just to keep people scared and quiet, he has another think coming. I'm going to tell everybody in this town some things I know about the sheriff and we'll see if he ever gets another vote. No, don't shush me, I mean it. I'm going to tell the people the truth!"

15

Opening the door to leave the courtroom the next morning, they heard the noise. There was a crowd outside two blocks long. Their own group had made signs, were passing out leaflets; the black newspaper had put out an issue this morning, with pictures of Leslie being carried to the car, the deputy's face as he beat her a contortion of hate.

The street was filled with marching and shouting and an occasional raised fist, but if there were a hundred women, there must have been over fifty strollers with toddlers inside—blue and red and brightly-decorated strollers, jingling their bells and rattling their plastic beads, each with one or two children laughing as if they were at a parade. The sky was overcast still but the temperature was back to fifty degrees. Some women carried brooms—twenty or so brooms weaving and thrusting in the air as the

147

people shouted, "Sweep the trash off the top." Another group was throwing something white over the sidewalks and streets and had, earlier, covered the steps to the jail.

The five were trying to hear what had happened since yesterday afternoon on the outside and tell their tale of the inside over the shouting and chants. Suddenly a noise and commotion turned everyone's head toward the jail steps. Someone had opened the fire hydrant standing a few yards this side; water gushed noisily into the streets. The pavement and sidewalk turned into foam and bubbles.

By the time the police had forced it closed again, the street was awash with soap suds. Billows of white foam rose up to the police car doors. Cars and officers seemed to be floating on a cloud. The police motioned the crowd back; they moved on the people so slowly to avoid slipping themselves that the adults watching laughed and the children clapped and jumped up and down.

"A rub-a-dub-dub," someone shouted and the children picked it up.

"The cops are cleaning up this town now."

" 'Pears to me they've overloaded the machine."

"Must have a whole lot of dirty wash."

"Get after that tattle-tale grey, boss!"

"Watch it you don't put the white in with the colored, boss. Colored runs."

"Used to. Color fast nowadays."

The women were all on the sidewalk opposite the jail. Suds covered the street, mounting over the sidewalk where the police were, declining with a slope and ending at the opposite sidewalk. A car appeared, moved slowly down the block, suds up over its wheels; its passage blew and scattered clumps of bubbles which drifted in the air like brief balloons. One landed on the hat of a police who knocked it away so vigorously na stirred up the suds at nan feet; a second clump detached itself and slowly rolled towards nan fellow officer. The group who had brought brooms began hitting suds from their side like balls over to the jail's side. The children threw what was left of the soap powder in their boxes high in the air like snow.

A fire truck clanged around the corner and pulled up in the middle of the suds, scattering them like feathers over the police. A fireman jumped down and began unwinding his hose, moving toward the hydrant.

"Don't do that, you fool!" a cop shouted. "There's a ton of detergent on the street."

"Tired? Irritable? Don't take it out on *him*."

"Look like he got the washday blues."

"Hey, firefighter, turn the hose on us!"

"Don't we get a bath over here? We're *dirty*."

"They got fourteen miracle ingredients in that soap."

"It'd take a miracle to get the stains out of this town."

"Easy on the starch now, chief. It'll rub your necks *red*!"

"Wonder is those guns drip-dry?"

"No, but they sure press easy. And permanent. Let's move."

The women were edging back toward the intersection; only a handful were still on the block when the police reached the middle of the street. They disappeared around the corner just as a loud clap of thunder shook the air and a sudden rain fell in torrents from the sky.

"This sure is gonna be some clean, white town."

"Us women and children are mighty grateful to you officers."

"All us average citizens is."

16

In private, the cook apologized to the carpenter for not being arrested also; she had felt she should take care of the children. "It must have been grim for you," the cook said. The carpenter thought she understood "grim;" she started to say . . . "I mean 'grim,' " the cook explained, "to be shut up in a cell with Three, since there would be too much temptation for you to let loose your hostility." The cook was lighting a cigarette and did not see the carpenter's face. "I know your relationship is based on hatred," the cook said. "I can understand that you need that—an outlet for your anger—but if I'd been there too I could have helped."

"Helped what?" The carpenter's voice was neutral in transition.

"Kept you from being too mean," the cook said. "To Three."

"I'm mean to Three?"

"I've seen it. I identify with Three. You've done the same thing to me, in the past." The cook's face was uncharacteristically still, set in points of definition.

The accusation sent the carpenter's mind back into a reinterpretation of her past; her imagination offered up a flood of faults. "Can't you give me an example?" she said.

"I heard you one night—you were speaking very loud and you know your voice is so . . . *positive*. You told Three she had to change. It was the way you said it. A demand. You were demanding that she change to . . . as if to suit you. Most people, if they love someone, try to accept them as they are, but you were . . . there was something in your voice that said you were going to force her to change."

"Oh." The carpenter was silent for several seconds.

"I felt I ought to tell you. You asked . . ."

"No, I'm glad you did. I was thinking." The carpenter frowned; her eyes as serious as noon sought the cook's. "If we're really involved with each other—any two people—don't we all change? Isn't that the point even?"

"Well, change comes. Sure, it happens. But it's different if you force someone."

"I'm not forcing Three. She is free . . ."

"It's your attitude. You're so positive, too strong—anyone would feel forced. I would."

"Did you?"

"Sometimes I started feeling forced and I resisted."

"You're sure it was me forcing you—not love or the relationship or something else?"

"I'm sure I felt it was you."

The carpenter touched her arm for a moment. "I'm sorry, I didn't mean . . ."

"Don't apologize!" The cook stood up and laughed

151

briefly. "We won't be able to talk at all if you're going to do that."

That night Stubby made an announcement: she was in love. The personal reason she had not joined in the take-over was that; she had spent the night with her new lover instead. The lover was not given a name; Stubby referred to it as "this person."

" 'This person' belongs to a group which is very political. They are organizing people all over the area around single issues and they are very effective. They have an office in Houston and an annotated mailing list and contacts and . . . I'll be working with them from now on. That's all I wanted to say."

Stubby was sitting back down when Sweeper rushed at her from the side and seized her in a congratulatory hug. "You're in love!" Sweeper said. "How marvelous—I'm so happy for you."

"You're really leaving?" Meredith said. "I'm sorry . . ."

"We'll have to learn Spanish ourselves," the cook said.

"I don't believe it," the carpenter said privately to Three. "It's too convenient."

"Well, I'm disappointed that she isn't a spy or at least a secret Trot," Three said. "But we can't trash na for falling in love."

"But to choose just that moment . . ." The carpenter's hands described a square in the air. "It sounds like she wanted an excuse. It's threatening, frightening, terrifying to be really close to twenty-five people— that intimate in an action where you're wrapped up in a room with all those others, so close . . . I know because I felt that last fall. You escape by choosing one person instead."

Three laughed. "My perfect harp! Can you work her back into a spy for me?"

The carpenter suddenly held Three's face. "Do you trust me?"

152

"I'm beginning to." Three's eyes were soft and serious. "You were fucking all right in that jail."

"You thought I'd bang on the bars and demand martinis?"

"If you want to know the honest truth, I thought you'd demand to be released and pay them, and then come back later with a lawyer for the rest of us."

"Tell me another truth: am I cruel to you?"

"I was such a battered child," Three said. "That I thought beatings were love. Therefore since you refuse to beat me . . ."

"I'm serious." The carpenter frowned. "As usual."

"I don't understand you then," Three said.

"I mean, do I force you to change? Force you at all? The carpenter explained, rephrasing the question, offering the example of the conversation the cook had overheard.

"I remember that night, sure," Three said. "There's another night I remember too, when I was about thirteen. We were spending the night with my cousins, all of us—I forget why. Us kids were in the only other room besides the kitchen; the grownups were talking in there. It was cold but there were nine of us lying on blankets on the floor, packed so tight we sure weren't cold—we were trading each other's air. Suddenly I felt I just couldn't stand it. I opened the window and climbed outside and sat in the outhouse. My mother found me when she came out to piss. I'd fallen asleep. She woke me up and I remember my teeth were chattering so I could hardly hear her—from fear as much as cold. I tried to tell her I couldn't stand it in that room with everybody on top of everybody else, and she gripped my shoulders hard to hold them still and said, 'You get back in there and stay there until you feel that crowd, until you feel crowded from your head to your toes, right down to the bone. And when you really feel it you're gonna make up your mind to do something about it.' I got back in the room and sat up till dawn listening to the other eight shuffling around

153

inhaling each other's exhales. The next day when
we got back home I went and got me a job at the
mill. That was where my head was at then: you
make some money and buy another room if you
can't stand being crowded. I wasn't old enough to
know anything else. But I sure learned that you
don't go out in the cold and freeze to death. My
goddamn angry parent, the only one I had any
respect for, made me learn that, forced me, if you
want." Three's arms hung loose and out to the
sides like a child's. "You remind me of her. You
have the same hands, knobby and square and always moving around. I used to know what she
was thinking by the way her hands moved, and
you're the same. I know when you're restless or
trying to be patient, or angry, or want to make
love. There's something about the set of your mouth,
too—my mother was serious all the time, like you.
She had to be, I guess."

The carpenter reached for Three's shoulders as
a way of occupying her knobby, square hands—
suddenly huge. "Maybe you can force me to learn
to laugh."

The city council discussed the problem of the
former Shadyside elementary school at its next meeting. They decided that it would be politic to offer
the building to a group who would put it to blame-
less use; it was clearly too tempting, standing there
empty and vulnerable. The Boy Scouts were chosen.

At the next meeting, it was discovered that the
Boy Scouts did not want the building. The vote
split was two to one to tear the building down.

Three brought the news back to the group.

"Tear it down?"

"And sow the ground with salt."

Sweeper lost custody of her children. Both sets

154

of grandparents agreed: she was too violent and unstable to be a parent.

"We're leaving this town anyway," Stubby said. "Sweeper can come with us."

"We're not leaving," Three said, her arm in the carpenter's. "We just started."

"Look," the cook said. "It's the egg woman!"

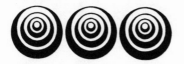

17

The carpenter stared out at the dawn, hypnotized like a comma on the plumbago bush whose blossoms were pale no-color now although the mind knew they were blue. The carpenter's eyes were suspended at the edge of the bush, waiting for increasing light to bring it into blue.

She was no longer the carpenter. Since jail, she had used the name her mother had given her at birth, possibly her real name. For six months she had called herself, and had lately been called by others, Henrietta. Henrietta—sometimes shortened to Rietta—had taken on a new sound, the sound of sound only: the "hen" which had humiliated her childhood with its connotation of silly maternity, the "etta" which pursued her adolescence like a weak rime for "get her," were now heard as an abstract combination of vowels and consonants, aurally harmonious, whose mood was merely

159

indicative. Henrietta: she was getting used to it like a face in a love affair.

She thought she saw blue on the plumbago bush—a trick of the mind. Under her determination to see sustained blue, the blossoms retreated back into no-color. Only the orange pail overturned in the grass was clearly orange.

She raised her eyes to the fence behind, spray-painted day-glo letters streaking "I love you, Harp" across the once-white boards.

"It's tacky, that's why you wince," Three had said after she put it there. She had sprayed her shoes and a spot on the carpenter's hand with the last sputter of the can. "It's blatant and loud—common—like me. It's for you to remember me by." She kissed the carpenter's hand and held its spatters to her cheek. "I have to go. You know that, don't you?"

The carpenter pulled Three's head to her shoulder and held her miniature body, stiff with departure. It was too late at night to scream and she knew too much to cry. She nodded. "You were leaving before you came. Ever since you got here, a little bit of you has been leaving week by week. I wonder there's enough of you left—or not left—to hold up your pants."

"Are you going to be the one person who understands me?"

"That's gonna be me. Woman to the bone and mother to the core. Never mind that my heart is breaking."

"Harp, don't say that."

Breaking? The carpenter held Three pressed against the place where the heart lived, heart now swollen into a throbbing weight aching against her chest, heart brought back to beating less than a year ago after a lifetime of ticks but already demanding that beating was its right.

"You stayed longer than I thought you would."

"Longer than I should have, you mean." Three pulled free and, taking the carpenter's hand in a last, deliberate

160

swing, turned them toward the house. "I really loved you though. Know that."

"If a river loves the land it passes through, you did."

"I'm no river, Harp," Three laughed. "More like a trickle."

"A rivulet, at least."

"Rivu*let*? Damn you."

The carpenter stopped just before the house and held Three's face for the last time. "It was the past tense that hurt."

Hurt like her lifelong recurring toothaches. Her tongue reached up to the left and felt there at the back molars the sure sore promise of a new bout with pain. Four times a year, as regular as the seasons, with the one in the spring sadistically the worst.

She had caught a cold during the week after jail and its virus, prone to attack the body's weakest spot, had aimed straight for her jaw, boring under the frayed gumline and into the bone to a safe hidden spot where it could wage its purest game of pain out of reach. Soft spongy frontline defense of gum, old porous lastline fort of crumbling bone, the carpenter knew that if her skull were ever found there would not remain enough of its lower portion to reconstruct even a conjecture of a jaw. The pain was quickly on a stampede, a million cattle running over a rotten fence. The carpenter had thought of money. Money bought dentists. But dentists had been bought for these vestigial teeth since they had first cut their way through infant gums; the carpenter's mouth had paid the rent for dentists in six cities and had given rise to the expression: put your money where your mouth is.

The carpenter's mouth throbbed with pain from her back jaw deep into her head . . . pain which by noon had fought and won against six aspirin and hourly doses of hot salt water, pain attacking the carpenter's will and undermining the will's resolve to get up once again and hold mouthful after mouthful of hot salt water against each aching side in turn, only hope of relief however minute. The carpenter fell back into pain, soaking her consciousness in the jab and throb which obliterated everything except itself.

"Can I get you an aspirin?" Three had said.

"An *aspirin*."

"You better go to the dentist. You look dead."

"Care is a myth. Fluoride and milk and fresh vegetables and checkups . . . all patriarchal distortions of some longlost opposite fact. I haven't eaten a piece of candy since I was ten, that's the trouble."

"Do you want an icepack?" Three said. "Or is a hot pack better?"

"You wouldn't know. I see." The carpenter turned her head into the pillow and groaned. Three hadn't even had a toothbrush as a child, now brushed her teeth erratically once or twice a week; still each time they came up white and sparkling like shells from the ocean, whole and eternal. "What's all this talk about dental care for the poor? It's a bill without any teeth in it. Forgive me, Three, I am down in the mouth today."

"I'm going to find you a woman dentist."

The carpenter groaned slowly to her feet and stumbled toward the bathroom's supply of hot water and salt. "*Any* dentist. The revolution sucks with toothless gums."

Henrietta had stayed in her room the morning Three left, only at the last minute going to the front window to watch her wave to the group who were glad to see her go. In the week that followed, the ache in Henrietta's heart soothed itself by listening to the others criticize Three. Each time a creak of pain started up again she sought out someone and let herself be oiled by a recitation of Three's faults. The supply of oil seemed endless.

After their failure to acquire the building, the health

project had set up an abortion referral service and women's health classes. The project thrived, women flocked to it, they were answering the telephone and counselling women from morning until late at night. But no sooner was it established and working well than Three began to push for more radical action. They were successfully helping women get abortions and understand their bodies. Hopefully they were also reaching them with the idea that their bodies were their own. Or was this, their sole project, Three challenged, by its emphasis defining women in terms of their reproduction function as usual? This is no revolution, it's social service, Three shouted. Most of the group applauded when Meredith shouted back that we can't even begin if someone is always going to disrupt.

But the carpenter knew that Three's departure owed nothing to the group's antagonism except timing. Three left because her blood only flowed when she was moving.

Henrietta too was beginning to feel like the salvation army, felt a restlessness every day that she tried to quiet by focussing on the few women who came to them as women wanting to understand. Most women came as adjuncts of their men. Too often the carpenter felt sure, with the young middle-class women, that they viewed the abortion as a denial of their choice— that they were being programmed for college and a good marriage and a baby would ruin their chances. The carpenter felt that some of them saw having a baby as the last way to rebel; others saw that the real reason they couldn't have a baby was that there was no way they could support it: the accusation, why don't you work on the sickness not the symptom? came from one angry woman. "I know," the carpenter said through the pain of total inadequacy and longed to escape. "But in the meantime . . ." Over half the women who came to them were black. The town chieftains, resisting pressure from Catholics and right-to-life groups, allowed the project to operate because they were preventing the birth of a certain number of blots.

Henrietta knew that Three was right but in the first week of her absence the carpenter's heart was filled with hate. She hated Three for leaving her a member of the group, one woman equal among many, vulnerable on all sides to friendships, requests for response, vague but ever-present possibilities of relationships with no guidelines of love; left her an object among objects to make her own way with no escape to a bed; left the days filled with people no more or less special than herself.

The carpenter was answering the telephone when a call came in from a young woman who spoke so faintly the carpenter could hardly hear her. "Can you speak any louder? Are you alone?"

"Just for a few minutes," the voice whispered. "They all went to the store for ice cream."

"They can't hear you until they get back," the carpenter said.

The woman was too terrified to speak in more than a loud whisper and the carpenter strained to hear. She was spotting . . . afraid she was going to miscarry. She was seventeen. The carpenter told her to meet her at the public hospital, gave her the address, asked her to name a time . . . eight tomorrow morning. "At the emergency entrance but don't go in. Meet me at the entrance to the driveway. Don't worry. I'm going to be your mother."

The next morning the carpenter walked up to two frightened-looking young women before she found Cathy. "Now look, you're not Cathy, your name is Chris and you're not seventeen you're eighteen. Try to remember your birthday: I wrote it down for you. You're old enough to go to the hospital without a parent but I'm a worried devoted mother, so call me Mom and don't be upset if I pat you or kiss your hand or stroke your forehead."

"We don't look alike," Cathy said.

"Sure we do." The carpenter felt they were in luck being the same race.

Cathy-Chris was dutifully admitted to emergency, wheeled around with her anxious mother following and patting, and her miscarriage attended to at eleven. The doctor came up to the carpenter. "You can go see her now. We've done a d. and c. She was miscarrying all right. You're her mother?" There was something in the doctor's face that showed he didn't believe it.

The carpenter went into the booth where Cathy lay. "He was awful," she whispered in tears. "He kept trying to make me admit I'd stuck something up myself. 'What'd you do it with?' he said. 'You might as well tell me, I'll find out anyway.' I didn't think he was going to treat me until I told him. But I didn't do anything, I really didn't, I kept telling him I didn't . . ."

"He said he did a d. and c.," the carpenter said. "Did he . . . scrape you out inside, I mean?"

"Finally. And he made me look at it . . ."

"Shhh, hush now, don't cry now. Let's get out of here."

"He said I have to stay here until Monday. I have to have a clean-out or something, and surgery closes at noon until Monday." She was shaking and the carpenter held her as if she were her own daughter. "I can't stay until Monday. My parents never let me stay out even with a girl friend."

The carpenter brought calm politeness up from the past and went back to the doctor. She began by telling him she was taking her daughter home and would bring her back on Monday. The doctor, flanked by his nurse, said, "I can order her to stay here. I don't believe you're her mother at all. No natural mother would endanger her daughter's health . . ."

Calm and politeness vanished without a trace. "She doesn't believe you're a doctor, for that matter," the carpenter said. "Bullying her and trying to make her admit a lie, threatening not to operate until she tells you she did something she didn't even do. No real

165

doctor would harass a patient if he really cared about her health." The carpenter brought out Chris's birth certificate and lay it in front of the nurse. "Here's her birth certificate."

They each read it with falling faces. "But this doesn't say the name of the mother," the nurse discovered triumphantly. "It doesn't say you're the mother."

"Look on the back," the carpenter said, and easily brought out proof that she was the mother named on the back.

Outside, the carpenter asked Cathy if she could come back to the house where their own doctor could tell them if there really was any further danger. Cathy agreed. "I'm really grateful to you," she said. "I shouldn't say this but I almost didn't call you. I'd heard you all were . . . lesbians, you know." Cathy lowered her eyes for a second as she said the word straight out. "But you're a mother." She laughed. "Isn't it amazing what people will say?" The carpenter was still thinking when Cathy said, "You're sure not like my mother though. I want to tell you something . . . you know how I got pregnant? I was raped."

"Good god," the carpenter said without thinking.

"I don't even have a boyfriend. I was coming home from babysitting and the car ran out of gas—I was only three blocks from home so I walked. A man pulled me into a bush and raped me." She made no attempt to say the word straight out; her voice shook. "He was . . . disgusting."

"Why didn't you tell your mother?"

"She wouldn't have believed me. She would have thought it was my fault. And she's told me time and time again to be sure and check the gas gauge on the car . . . it was my fault."

"Your fault for being raped? It's his fault—if that's word enough for it, the pig."

"Mother would have thought I enticed him or something." Her voice began to shake again. "I know

166

she wouldn't have believed me. I know."

"Okay. I believe you. Look, you must be hungry. Want to stop for a hamburger?"

Cathy shook her head. "I couldn't eat. It still hurts, down there. I have money for a hamburger, I just don't want one." She started to fumble in her purse; brought up two dollars. "See? I have money. I'm just not hungry."

The carpenter stumbled over the open yard, aiming for the willow tree, composing an angry mind-letter to Three. Dear Three. Saint Three. She accused the moon over the willow tree, a ring of haze around its high half-circle like a ring of politics around its heart. Dear Saint Three. I see your halo very well. Is Cathy male because her hair is teased? You'd like to beat this willow to the ground because it weeps, because it won't stick its feathers in the air and make them knives . . . would you say its tracery entices? Take your wild deer face and run your anger, ride your truth until lather makes it white but don't look down—that's lipstick on the road not blood and some spilled toe-nail polish on the sheet. I could squeeze your bright red heart until it spurted and collapsed and not relieve one hand's hate, my heart's hate, I hate you Three. Dear Pure. Dear Uncompromised. Lies are truth where truth is not believed.

A moving, panting stumble through bushes was the cook, gasping, "It's Sweeper . . . I have to get my breath . . . wait . . ." She took the carpenter's hand, gripping it. "Sweeper's back. She's hysterical. I need your help."

When they reached the house, Sweeper was standing in the front door screaming at a man who stood outside on the porch. A woman stood behind him.

"You can't come in! Go away!"

"I'm a friend," the woman said. "He's her lawyer. We're trying to help her."

"She says you can't come in," Carter said. "So you

can't."

"Just let me explain," the man said.

"Who is he, Sweeper?"

"I'm her lawyer. I'm trying to help her and she gets into a crazy fit . . ."

"Pig!"

"He's my lawyer all right," Sweeper screamed through the screen at the man. "He says he's going to get my children back but all he does is talk. I'm going to go get them myself . . ."

"If you do that no one can help you, you fool," the man said. He appealed to Carter. "Just let me explain . . ."

The cook explained to the carpenter: the man and woman weren't here before, just Sweeper who had come in begging for a car, she was going to kidnap her children, no one was helping her . . .

"I thought Stubby and her new pals were . . ." the carpenter stopped. "Why didn't they get her a woman lawyer?"

Sweeper shut the door and leaned with her back against it, facing the group. She was breathing in rushes and her eyes were glittering but she made an effort to speak slowly and calmly. "Let me tell you the whole thing now," she said. "Just let me tell you the truth and then you can decide if I'm right or not. Stubby and the other women were going to help me . . . fight this injustice as they put it, and they were real sympathetic and I thought they were angry too, so they got this lawyer and he told me he wanted to help me but he said it would take time and could I be patient. I said I'd try. I talked to him all one morning, the other women were there, and he looked real pleased and said he'd start working on it right away. But after that every time I tried to talk to him, just call him on the phone, he was always out. The other women said it took time and in the meantime it would help to make some speeches and talk to newspapers . . . help me and help other women in the same boat. So I did. I first

168

told a big group just how my parents and my ex-husband's parents had never liked me and how my ex-husband would do anything to get back at me which is how he came to talk them into getting that court order to get custody of the kids after we were in jail. Because he's the meannest bastard alive. Well, after that talk the women explained to me that it wasn't my husband personally it was the system that made this happen and I didn't have the right emphasis. I said I was just telling the truth—he *is* the meannest bastard alive. Well, they said could I tell more about the building we were setting up and the day care and health services and how they'd put us in jail, because then it looked like they took my kids because I was trying to fight injustice and all. And I said, sure, because I thought that building was the greatest thing that ever came down the pike. But I felt funny saying that because I was just along, I hadn't thought up any of it, I was just there because I didn't have any place else to go or any way to look after my kids while I was at work. It didn't sound natural for me to be saying all the things they said I should say. But I said some of them and then they asked would I just as soon wear an everyday dress instead of getting so dressed up every time we spoke, and I said no, it shows respect for people when you get dressed up if you're going to appear on a stage and I wouldn't feel right unless I wore the best dress I had. But it wasn't just my dress. Last night I heard them making fun of my glasses—these glasses. They were laughing about how they turned up in points with little glittery things on them and how they bet I thought princesses wore glasses like these and how were they going to deal with these people's royal fantasies. That's when I told them they didn't have to. I told them that the real fantasy was that I ever thought they were more than a royal pain in the ass. Excuse the expression but that's what I said."

Sweeper was interrupted by shouts and hugs and

"right on's" from the women in the room.

"Let her finish," Andy said. "I want to hear the story."

"Shhh."

"Go on, Sweeper."

"That's all. I left. I was so mad I was muttering to myself on the bus all the way down here from Austin. The kid sitting next to me changed seats with his mother, I was muttering so I scared him. But every time I thought about the abortion rallies I'd talked at and the reporters I'd told my story to and how for two months I'd been talking and appearing and not getting one iota closer to my children . . . I'd get so mad I couldn't see straight. I decided I'm going to go get the children myself. They must think I'm nothing, just a miserable piece of nothing not to have come after them by now."

By one o'clock that night Sweeper's two children were safely tucked into Stubby's former bed and sound asleep.

"It was so simple," Carter said. "I stood watch while Sweeper opened a window screen and in less than five minutes was back with the two kids, half asleep, one holding each hand and quiet as mice. They won't even miss them until morning."

"We talked to a lawyer. Jane. She said, 'Good god, you didn't!' She said she'd be down Saturday. She also said to get them out of here."

"Sweeper wants to go to Florida."

"Florida?"

"Yeah. She thinks she'd like Florida."

"Do we know anyone in Florida? What about California?"

"New York is the obvious place."

"That's no place to raise kids."

"They don't have to be raised there. They can stay there until Sweeper wins them back. New York judges always . . ."

Sweeper came back into the room. "She's got to be the greatest lawyer that ever walked the face of the earth," she said with a huge grin.

"And she's coming down the pike," Nicky said.

"Then she's got to be the greatest lawyer that ever came down the pike," Sweeper laughed. "I can't help it, I'm beaming from ear to ear."

"What'd she say?"

"She said I have to stay in town if I want to win the court fight but to hide the children."

"This is the first place they'll look."

"Come on, let's think. We only have until morning."

"We don't have that long if the father-bastard gets home really drunk tonight and goes in to stare at those sweet sleeping babies so he can cry himself to sleep," Sweeper said. "He wasn't there. Just his folks."

"How can we hide two kids in a town like this?"

"We could if they were black," Leslie said.

By ten the next morning Leslie had cut two Afro wigs down to child size and Meredith was mixing make-up. "It's too bad it's so hot," Meredith said. "If it was winter we could just darken their hands and faces."

The children watched solemnly. "Now let's rehearse," Leslie said to the two little girls. "When you hear me run up sounding real mad and saying, 'Come on right now, we're going to be late to the clinic,' that means the play has begun. Now in this play I pretend to be your mama. We run and jump in the car and dash away to see the reindeer and eat ice cream. Now you don't say *any*thing after I start running up pretending to be mad. Just remember that I'm supposed to be your mama and everyone's watching."

"Is this dark enough?" Meredith said.

"The cops are going to have to be really dumb to fall for this anyway," the carpenter said. "Maybe we ought to make them boys."

"And cut my babies' hair?" Leslie knelt to apply

dark to the older girl's face. "Now if we're really good everyone may want to see us do it again. I tell you what. The second time you can scream and kick and cry and play like you don't want to go and I'll pick you up and put you in the car. Would you like that? You can make the biggest fuss you know how . . . just so you don't get yourself scared."

"I'm not scared," the child said. Her sister's blue eyes were round with wonder and she shook her head, "Me not 'cared."

Leslie laughed. "You know something? I think you're the greatest little girls that ever came down the pike."

Sweeper came by after work and gasped when she saw her children, who were following Leslie everywhere. She said quickly, "Why they look darling. I've always said Negro children were the cutest."

"Sweeper!" Meredith said.

"It gets worse," Leslie said. "I'm really digging being their mama."

"Wasn't this whole thing done in a Shirley Temple movie?" The carpenter saw that none of them were old enough to remember.

"That's why it'll work!" Sweeper's voice was angry in fear.

"It'll just have to," Leslie said.

The cook was working on a painting in the driveway. The carpenter had not been able to talk to her since Three left except through a ring of alarm clocks around her mind. Today the carpenter was depressed in a way which brought back her whole past . . . depression and gloom settled like coal dust in the crevices of her brain for the first time since she had joined the movement.

She watched the cook work and thought that that was it: while she herself had been chasing after a fantasy of being whole the cook had slowly worked through food to art. The carpenter could no longer hate Three and where the hate had raged and died a vacuum sucked

172

in on all surfaces of her soul: if Three had used her to get control over "upper classness" by loving and then throwing her away, the carpenter had equally used Three to take care of her own class guilt; where Three had been motivated by childhood envy, the carpenter's own life was dictated by fashions in the movement. In the still ice of her present vacuum, the carpenter felt that she could never feel again but her mind promised that if she did, it (mind) could be counted on to call that feeling spurious, to remember and destroy. Because she was aware of a tiny glimmer, an excitement at seeing the cook's concentrated back every inch of which the carpenter knew the feel of . . . she refrained from even thinking the words, by heart.

Henrietta connected the garden hose and turned it on. A gentle droop of water, all their pressure could provide in this month of water shortage, was warm and adequate. She held the hose end close beneath the plumbago bush, up against its stalk hidden by blue and green.

It was the day Three left, Mother's Day, that she had planted the bush—to celebrate fertility not commercialism, she told everyone. And to keep her mind from remembering Three's glowing face from the night before when they had spray-painted all the plate glass in town displaying mother pacifiers. Three's face, laughing with the release mischief provided, had made no connection with the carpenter's awkward smile, her stiff arm trying to enjoy smearing, her fear of being caught at something so unsuitable for her age. Three was celebrating the end of a liberated love-affair and the carpenter's prepolitical smile was like the hard tense back of a rejected child, rejecting back.

The plumbago bush was small and overpriced and wrapped in rose tinfoil but the blue of its sparse blossoms was the blue of pearls if pearls were blue. Only the cook had not been fooled. "That's called the vegetation cure," the cook whose name was Audrey had said. "My grandmother used to do that. She'd

173

grow flowers in her Brooklyn window and sit and look at them all afternoon as if the room behind her didn't exist."

Henrietta lost interest in the plumbago bush when she began to see that her hatred of Three came from her own terror of being one of the crowd. She began to analyse the terror, she intruded the subject of fear of the group into every group, she found she could relate to each member of the group separately and safely by discussing her fear. But she watered the plant dutifully just the same, caring for it as if to protect it from the knowledge that she no longer cared for it. It throve. It wasn't supposed to do that; it was supposed to respond to love not efficiency. But it grew and blossomed and was now fat with tiny pure-blue blossoms.

She propped the hose in a forked bottom twig and let the waste of water dribble unheld. A stream came over the saturated dirt; she moved her foot into it and stared at the pale patches the water made between her dusty toes. A sudden gust of hunger made her long for a cigarette for the first time in a year. Her hands stripped off a twig from the bush and pushed bits of mud into mounds. Her mind went out of focus. Because she could no longer feel love of Three. Or hatred. Her memory dutifully reported that she had loved her. It was no longer even important whether she believed it or not. The sounds of her heart were beginning to resemble ticks again, the barely audible tchk-tchk of a ladies' watch.

The cook did not want to look at the carpenter; her eyes were fresh from dreams of a baby with an ugly old face turned up to her for washing, an indestructible rubber face that clung still to the inside of her eyes as a thing so far on the other side of beauty that she knew she would never know beautiful again except there. But the carpenter's face was across the table, low on her slumped shoulders so that it was level with the cook's

174

own; the cook's eyes, reluctantly starting upward, stopped at the hands which were twisting a torn beer-label into a paper snake.

"I've missed you."

The cook felt the words spring across at her like a pair of claws gripping their prey. "We've known each other too long not to feel absence," the cook said, her own words sliding from her mouth like steel tape.

The carpenter's hand lay unnaturally still on the formica, as if told to see how long it could just sit quietly. The cook stared at it—a well-behaved lump. Staring, the cook felt the hand would burst if it could not move; would, if it did move, seize the cook's hand and mash and knead the two hands together until their separate outlines disappeared, until they were worked like clay into a single . . . hand, if need be.

Abruptly the carpenter stood up and, her hand gripped into a fist at her side, walked over to the bar to ask the man there to turn the television down. He stared at her for several seconds and shook his head.

"Let's change booths," the carpenter said, picking up both bottles and glasses.

At the new booth, five feet farther away from the language of baseball, the cook looked suddenly at the carpenter's face. "Did I tell you I got a letter from the children's father?" the cook said, pretending an English absentmindedness, this beer a daily tea.

"Tom? When would you have told me?"

"It was a totally new letter for him. A change." The cook took a deep dive into her logic. Everything swung on the phrase, "hatching the hate in my own nest." A strange phrase for Tom. Not at all typical? The carpenter nodded agreement. And began to be interested. If he saw himself as hatching this hate, did that mean it would soon be busting out of its egg and leaving the nest? Or did he mean he'd been sitting on his hate and was now going to admit it—let it out to speak or cheep or something? Or did he mean the nest was now crowded with hate, hate with its mouths open taking up

175

all his energies?

"All those things," the cook said, unable to see contradictions. "He especially mentioned how he sometimes hated you. As well as me. Sometimes more than me although not, he said, as regularly."

"Were we competing for Tom's hate?"

"His hate . . . facing his hate is a very important thing for him to do. But it was the word hatching that was so unbelievable. The word means only one thing: Tom is thinking of himself as a parent instead of a child for the first time."

The passive of hatching—being warmed from above while wrapped in hardening albumin (white)—was also important, the cook thought out loud. But some people don't need that. The carpenter's hand had returned to motion, picking at the beer label now limp with damp. "You're very strong," the cook said, looking directly into the carpenter's face. Sun came into the darkened airconditioning through a gap in the abstract curtains, slicing the carpenter's face; three-quarters of it was bleached like an over-exposed photograph, a fading memento of what someone wanted to remember. The cook offered a gentle, flirtatious smile. "I've always thought of you as strong. You are. Even when you are not feeling strong at the moment."

The carpenter got up to pull the curtain's gap off her face and brought them each another beer. The cook re-adjusted to a shaded face, felt as a loss the removal of that sun-washed paleness. Her mind stuck at the base of her tongue. If I had words, she thought, I could ask simply, what's the matter? If I knew simple grammar and could ask anything simply. If I had not been taught too well that to ask is simply rude. If I ask complexly . . .

"Have you heard from Three?"

The carpenter shook her head, slipped her eyes away from the cook's face and attached them onto the pocket-sized music selector now receiving a meaningless shaft of sun.

I got a letter from her this morning, the cook thought, clamping her teeth around the thought. I got a letter from her . . . I got a letter . . . I will not say a simple or complicated word, the cook said sternly to herself, smoking through the long silence. "I got a letter from her this morning," the cook said. The carpenter's face flicked open and closed like a camera shutter. "It was just a note asking for an address . . . nothing personal. Almost a postcard. She asked about you." The cook's hand, wanting to reach for the carpenter's, stopped at the ashtray and pushed the lit tobacco into the ashes until it was out and very out and after. "I won't mention you if you don't want me to."

The carpenter leaned forward, her face as pale, her skin as thin as smoke against a cloud—transparent waves of energy directed at the cook's helpless eyes. "Would you believe me if I told you I loved you?" the carpenter said.

"Do you believe you?" The cook's voice was crisp. Love is all those awkwardly-printed words on mother's day cards that we taught them, because we couldn't bear to hear them say, I eat your soul because I must grow big and replace you. Love is that word sticky with semen which we begged them to say instead of, Stand still, target. Love is the grasp of drowning arms onto drowning arms as we push each other under.

"What time is it?" the cook said.

"Let's have one more beer," the carpenter said. "The ball game isn't even over."

Incoherent energy launched the cook into paragraphs of words, which sometimes paralleled her thoughts and sometimes replaced them. She talked of hatching and what eggs meant. She was an artist. The nest, any nest, scratched. She was leaving the group because the group wanted her nest and she was letting them have it. But she was taking her nest with her, her own three bleeding mouths because now Tom looked like he wanted them. If he didn't want them she would have let him have

177

them; wanting, he is monstrous. He would raise them.
Then she would succeed. She would force open gallery
doors. She would play any game necessary. Art was
only politics, she had learned with that flesh left her,
and her own insanity could be sold. "It's not selling
out, it's selling in," she said.

"Come live with me," the carpenter said.

Two people can't do that, the cook was certain. One
would want an ashtray emptied and the other would
grow irritated at that constant emptying of ashtrays.
Besides, there is no reason to live together any more.
She had just learned that she could be alone. Cooking
was the language she used with people; she had no more
gifts. "You have always been too strong to be seduced
by cooking."

The carpenter, fairly sober, rattled off the things she
could cook . . . oendaw, hush puppies, chicken and
tamale pie.

"I have nothing left to give," the cook said. She
laughed. The carpenter was going to ignore the laugh.
The cook added, "Especially to a blonde."

The carpenter was speaking so clearly that the cook
trembled. She felt coherence wrapping around her like
a blanket. The inside of the blanket was talking about
sharing, not those other kinds of love; the love the
carpenter meant was like fertilizer, like the brick house
for the third pig, like singing a song together even
though one of them couldn't carry a tune. It was
carrying each other's tunes. The carpenter wanted her
tune carried. She spoke of money, offered a working
week of bookcases, walls, custom-made cabinets. She
said, We can talk about the ashtrays or throw them at
each other. The cook wished the carpenter would get
drunker; clarity was making her blink, blind. The carpenter reached for her hand instead. The cook, instantly
imagining the bartender watching . . . calling the
police, snatched her hand away.

It would have to be done with words. I am alive
only when I am with you. Your separate being is as

178

precious to me as a character I am loving in a novel. We are below power and can trust one another. "I hate these words," the carpenter said.

The cook tried to be reasonable in words. If we didn't each have so many children, if there were just two of us, if we could go off somewhere, if society were different . . . but as things are, it's hopeless. You must know that.

The carpenter laughed and paid their check. "Let's go," she said. She felt like doing a dance. She was going to sing—to hell with tunes.

Outside, the heat made them gasp. "When I was growing up," the carpenter said. "Teenage girls held hands with each other on their way to the movies. I hated it. I wish we were teenage girls now, in dresses." Two elderly women met and kissed in front of the town's best restaurant; disappeared inside, one touching the other's shoulder. The carpenter took the cook's hand and swung it to a teenage rhythm before the cook pulled away. "Your telling me how strong I am is beginning to make me feel strong. Now all we have to do is change society," the carpenter said, kissing the air beside the cook's face.

It was blue. The carpenter stared. Blue remained. A hidden bird sang startlingly close to her ear and she jumped. The light was certain now; the blue was strong and sustained and for all its paleness, unmistakably blue. It was time to wake the cook.

She turned to the bed. The sheet covering the body there rippled under the ceiling fan making the body appear to be slightly moving in bizarre quivers. The head was hidden beneath a pyramid of two pillows. She picked up one pillow, uncovering hair; she picked up the other pillow.

"It's time to go," she said to the face of her love.

The children were waiting in the car. The carpenter stepped over five bodies in sleeping bags rolled

179

out on the living room floor—women who had arrived last night to take their places. Chris followed her to the car.

"Sure you don't want to come?"

Chris shook her head. "I'll stay."

"Goodbye, darling."

"Goodbye, Mom."